Unlocking
Your
Self-Healing
Potential

Josef Ulrich is an anthroposophical therapist at the Öschelbronn Clinic in Germany with many years' experience of working with people at different stages of health and illness, in particular those with a cancer diagnosis.

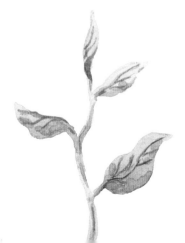

Unlocking Your Self-Healing Potential

A journey back to health
through creativity, authenticity
and self-determination

Josef Ulrich

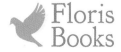

Floris
Books

Disclaimer

The ideas and suggestions in this book are intended for use alongside medical treatment. Readers with health issues should always consult medical professionals. The author and publisher do not accept any liability.

Translated by Matthew Barton

First published in German as *Selbstheilungskräfte:*
Quellen der Gesundheit und Lebensqualität by Aethera in 2016
First published in English by Floris Books in 2018
© 2018 Josef Ulrich

Josef Ulrich has asserted his right under the
Copyright, Designs and Patent Act of 1988 to be
identified as the Author of this Work

 Also available as an eBook

British Library CIP data available
ISBN 978-178250-533-4
Printed by Great Britain
by Bell & Bain, Ltd

For Jana-Anastasia, Bill, Lillian, Anna-Lena, Luca and Elliott
and for Anna-Jäel, Holger and Elisa;
for you, for me

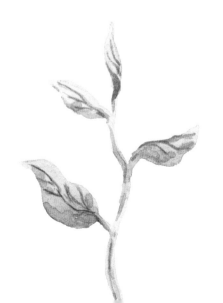

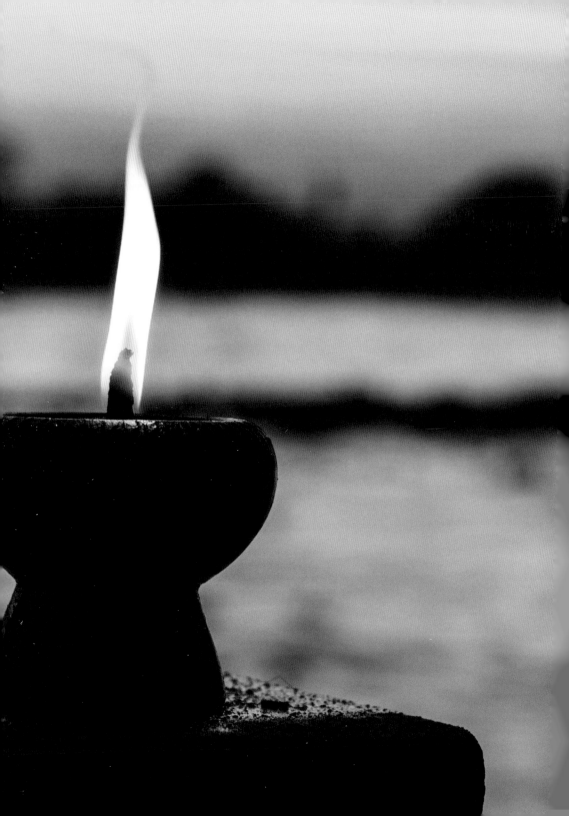

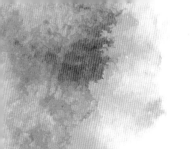

Contents

Foreword

Do we have self-healing capacities? Of course. We all know that a wound or broken bone can heal up by itself. But what about everything else between skin and bone – inside each cell of the body? Are self-healing forces at work there too?

Yes indeed. Without these regenerative powers, we would soon die, as all our cells are constantly being damaged in smaller and larger ways. They are damaged and then our bodies repair or replace them.

So how can we best support our healing potential?

Some answers to this feel certain. We know that vital elements of the healing process include our will to live, belief in our capacity to heal and a loving connection with life.

But, you may ask, how can the will kindle the flame of my healing energy? How can I maintain a belief in healing when life's unfathomable potential is limited to current finite human knowledge? How can love unfold its power in me when I am confronted daily by events that cast great doubt on the good in human beings? We all continually see how greed and lust for power cause natural and human devastation across the world.

Each subjectively oriented human being carries the power to foster processes of healing at every level. I believe we can all find within ourselves a loving presence of mind; perception of the other; true meaning; authentic feelings; valid decisions – and the capacity to act upon them. And we can cultivate these qualities throughout our lives. We are not victims but co-creators of the human world around us.

Each of us can start with ourselves. We can begin to live the change we wish to see, and *you* can live it in your own body, self and life.

When we are threatened by grave illness, the inner artist of our lives can be re-awoken; the inner navigator of our soul, shining at the core of our being, can reassert a luminous power. There are many people who, in illness, find their path and pursue it, often gaining health in the process, even when, from a medical perspective, their situation had seemed irrecoverable.

The ideas contained in this book are based on my conversations with many different patients as they journeyed through life-threatening illness. They shared the discoveries and insights that came to them in times of great personal difficulty. I hope their experiences will help my readers rekindle their own powers of self-healing, and follow where they lead.

Josef Ulrich

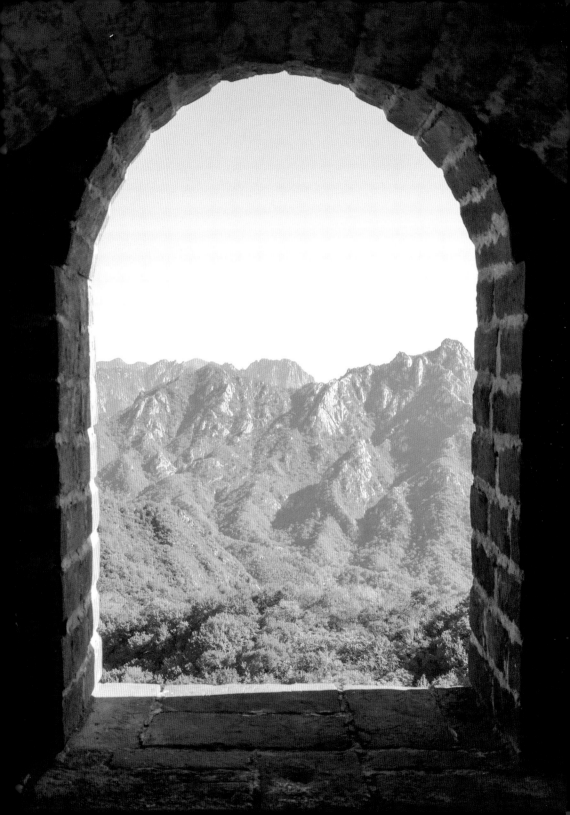

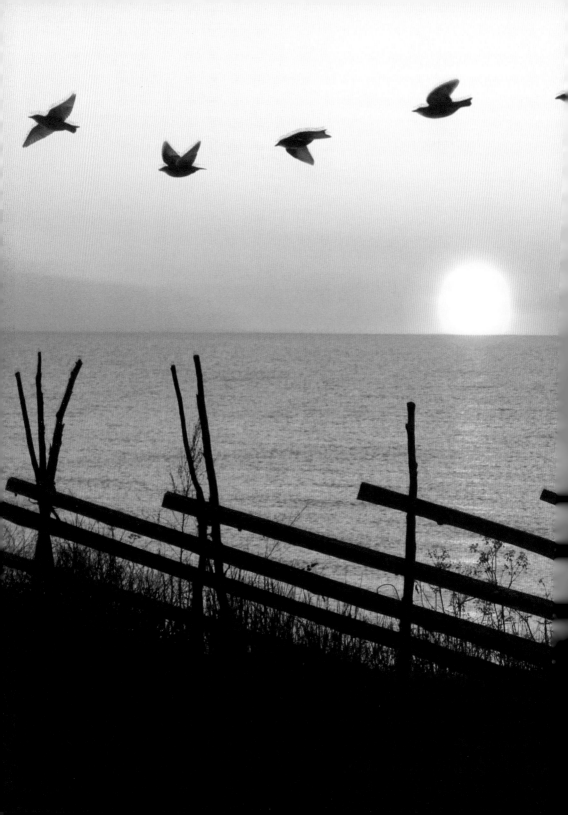

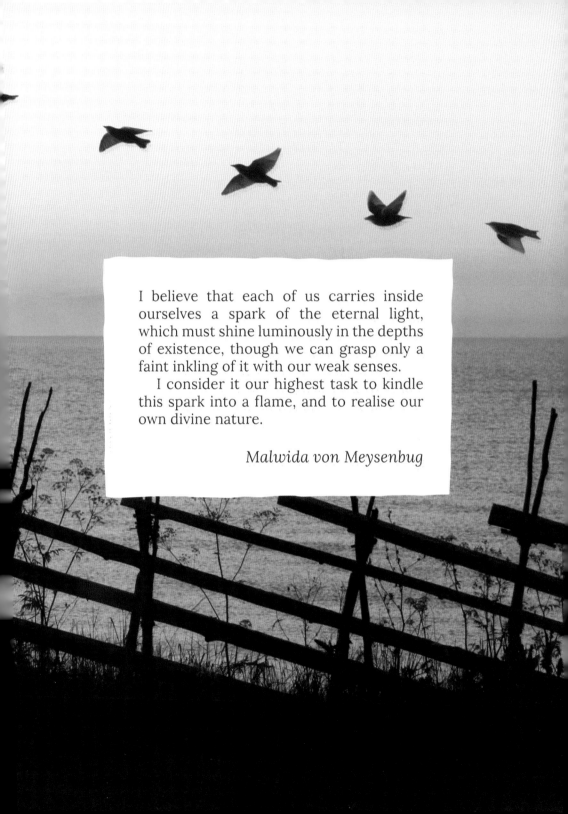

I believe that each of us carries inside ourselves a spark of the eternal light, which must shine luminously in the depths of existence, though we can grasp only a faint inkling of it with our weak senses.

I consider it our highest task to kindle this spark into a flame, and to realise our own divine nature.

Malwida von Meysenbug

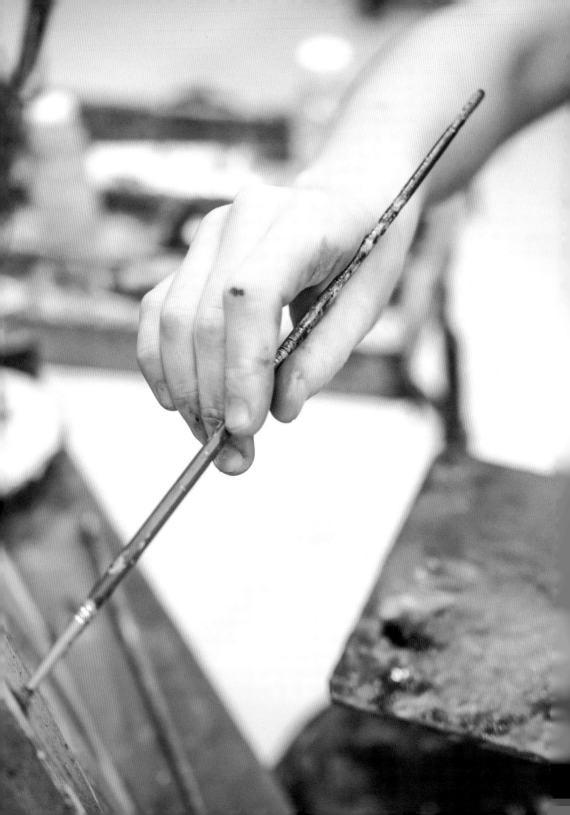

Introduction

In my work as an art therapist, I have often met people who have suffered a life-threatening illness that, astonishingly, does not end as predicted. During their illness these people often seem to develop a striking degree of creativity.

Creativity and the immune system

Thirty years ago, these meetings led me to wonder whether there might be a connection between a person's creativity and the strength of their immune system, between their inner being and their body's life forces. Do processes of the psyche have an affinity with those of the immune system? Was it possible, I wondered, that an authentic and self-determined life could act as a 'model' for the immune system, thus preventing illnesses or supporting their cure? Perhaps authenticity and self-determination could unlock powers of self-regeneration we never even dream of, by directing people back to the originating, intrinsic impulses underlying their lives?

My experience now tells me this is so. I believe people develop special capacities as they engage in stages of the creative process.

Triumph of the human spirit

People in crisis situations report that their mental or spiritual outlook enabled them to survive. Victor Frankl, as we know, found in the concentration camp where he was incarcerated that ultimate freedom resides in our inner stance toward whatever situation we face.[1]

Despite 27 years of imprisonment, Nelson Mandela never succumbed to hatred or the desire for revenge. He used this time to work toward the goal of peaceful co-existence in South Africa. For many years he kept recalling and repeating the poem 'Invictus' by William Ernest Henley,[2] the two last lines of which read: 'I am the master of my fate, I am the captain of my soul.' Mandela made these lines a living reality for himself, developing the strength to be master of his thoughts, to manage his feelings without letting rancour or violence take hold in his heart.

Another well-known figure is the British physicist and astrophysicist Stephen Hawking, who contracted amyotrophic lateral sclerosis. Despite a body that had been more or less unviable for decades, he developed an extraordinary power of mental activity, which sustained him for decades and gave his vivid, humorous spirit a dwelling.

The patient is the key to healing

Modern medicine, which has proven of inestimable value in many fields, has nevertheless given rise to the idea of patients as passive 'victims' of their illness. Disease is portrayed as giving rise to symptoms that must be medically suppressed or eradicated. Holding these assumptions, it is easy to lose sight of the patient as an active and vital contributor to their cure.

What is creativity?

Some readers, on hearing this talk of creativity, might well think that it is not one of their gifts. Many patients come to my art therapy sessions convinced they cannot paint. But in fact, this bears no relation to life's reality. As so often, a fixed idea about ourselves intrudes and paralyses possibilities. The potential for creativity in every single person means simply that anyone can shape and configure their world. As Albert Steffen puts it:

> To be an artist in this sense is possible for all people in every walk of life as long as they themselves grasp the transformative initiative. This does not have to be by using material substance formed into an artwork, or words, or music, or colour. It can also be a friendship, a work relationship, an illness, a misfortune or a blow of fate. Nothing is beyond reach of the artistic impulse, oneself least of all. Accordingly, being an artist means becoming fully human in the truest sense.[3]

Creative forces do not have to be expressed on paper. What I do with my patients could be called 'art therapy in the mind'. In our minds we paint our thoughts, concerns and anxieties, as well as our intimations of joy, our confidence and trust. By so doing we are co-creators of the reality we experience. Our thoughts have a decisive effect on how our life develops, and often also on the course of an illness.

A patient is more than an illness

Health and illness are both always present inside us. Over the last thirty years I have been privileged to meet thousands of patients, and while many of them, in the view of medicine, had the same condition, the same diagnosis, each and every one of them had their own particular path and journey. I met people whom doctors believed should no longer be alive, let alone able to recover, while others suddenly and unexpectedly died. And there were people who died happily and with gratitude in their hearts, whereas for others it seemed very difficult to let go and find peace. I can assure you that each of them was more than their illness: each one was, and is, a human being.

If every person who had a CAT scan was given a print-out of all their cells, they would see a tangible picture of the fact that they have many more healthy cells in their body than sick ones.

Besides our illness, we still live as a whole person with our healthy outlooks, feelings and abilities. I suppose you could say that my work has involved me specialising in working with the healthy aspect of a patient. Patients and I work together to make what is healthy still healthier, so that they can recover.

This book is based on notes from seminars and discussions with people who were facing a life-threatening disease. The thoughts expressed here arose largely in such discussions or seminars, so patients themselves have played a great part in the book. I want to thank them all, several thousands of them, for their openness, their questions, their quests and their struggles.

Finding your healing path

I would like to think that this book might give you the courage and trust to pursue your own individual path and that, whatever happens in your life, you find all the help that you need.

My aim is to support you in learning what will help you unfold your full, self-regenerative potential, to find ways to integrate this into your life, or in other words to overcome obstacles and hindrances, and perhaps to gain a sense of the meaning of your illness and of the challenge it has brought to you.

Reading the book, with its rich store of life experiences, might be seen as a journey. Welcome aboard! Our trip should lead us toward a healthier kind of thinking, one which helps us to support our own regenerative forces. On this voyage we will be taking three helpful guiding lights.

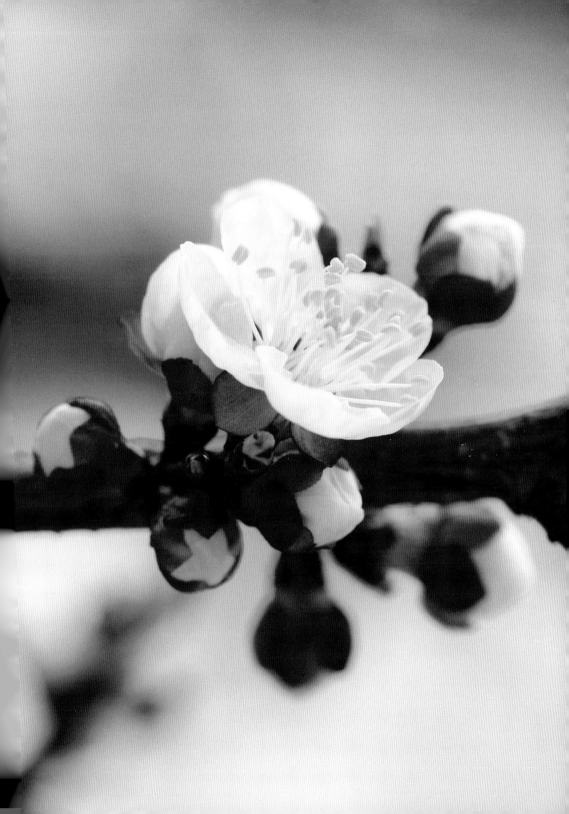

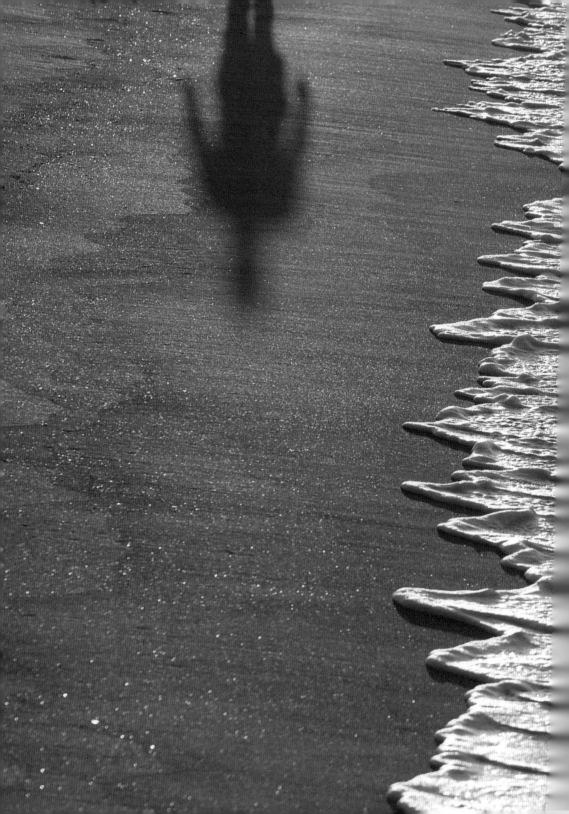

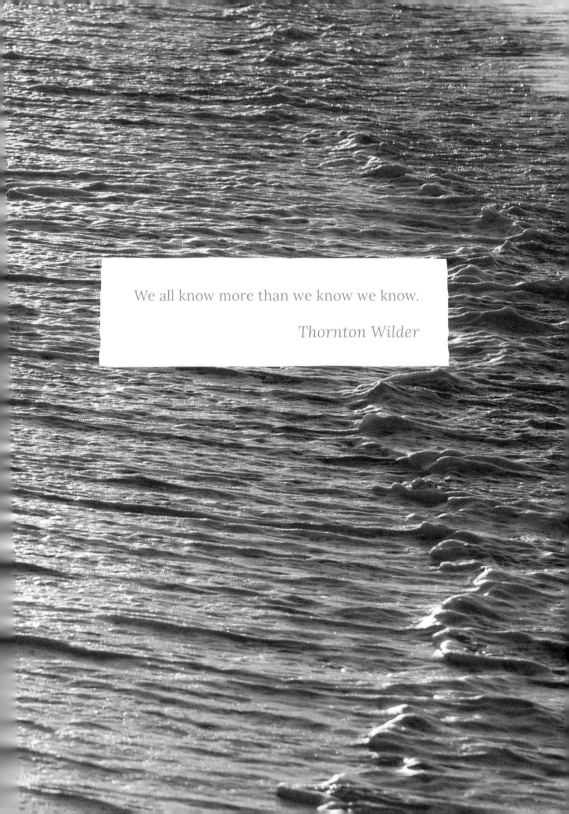

We all know more than we know we know.

Thornton Wilder

Three
Guiding Lights

On this journey towards greater self-healing potential, you will carry a small rucksack containing three helpful guiding lights: your healthy common sense, openness to possibility and also your own inner physician.

Healthy Common Sense

Whatever you may have read, heard or seen, whatever you have studied and learned, your true knowledge goes far beyond it. You know a great many things without having studied them – they are simply there for you as inner certainty.

And when you set out to strengthen your self-healing powers, please always attend to what your healthy common sense is telling you. Try to sense its loving support as you seek to rediscover your potential, your own store of experience, wisdom and knowledge.

Untreatable versus incurable

Many of us have an inner sense that the fact an illness is medically *untreatable* does not inevitably mean that it is *incurable*. The soundness of this intuition is shown by 'spontaneous remissions'. These do not happen often, but they do happen. Patients recover even when this outcome was wholly unexpected and remains medically inexplicable.[4]

Openness

The second guiding light that will be helpful on your journey is 'openness to reality'.

In modern, highly specialised fields of medicine it is easy to find professionals with different points of view, some of whom may think that their perspective is the only correct one. This does not cultivate openness, or insight.

More than flesh and blood

Openness involves becoming aware that we human beings are more than a material conglomeration measurable in kilos and centimetres. Being open to reality is to acknowledge that we are more than biochemical processes. If human life were a purely physical, material thing, the placebo effect could not happen, and only a 'real' medicine would work.

I want to invite you to attend to what a quiet voice within may already be telling you, and to be open to the possibility that, more than flesh and blood, you are a being constituted of body, soul and spirit.

A story: Paracelsus and the six diagnoses

Six physicians stand before a corpse and discuss what the patient died of. The first thinks it was the *cholera bacillus*. The second objects that many have been infected with it but did not die, and says that the main cause of death was the patient's weak immune system and poor vitality. The third physician says that, knowing the patient to be full of anxiety, she thinks that he attracted the cholera to him, as it were, and so his mental state was the real cause of death. The fourth physician claims to have known the patient even better, and says he was cowardly and lacked courage, was unable to make any decision, and so ultimately his weak ego was responsible for his deterioration. The fifth physician, surveying what all the others have said, decides that taking all these factors together it is clear that it was the patient's destiny to die, for otherwise all these things would not have conspired against him as they did.

And now the five physicians turn expectantly to the sixth and ask to hear his opinion.

Imagine that you are this sixth physician. I invite you to give your opinion. Which of the five others do you think was right? Was it the physical fact of the *cholera bacillus*, the patient's poor vitality, his anxious and fragile emotional state, his general lack of resolve, or his destiny?

The sixth physician was Paracelsus himself. In the story what he says is: 'Each of you is right in what you affirm, and each of you wrong in what you repudiate!'

Paracelsus is telling us to maintain openness: do not get tied to a single perspective rejecting all others, as they may have equal validity.[5]

The Inner Physician

The third guiding light is always by your side. This is the 'inner physician' in each one of us.

No one knows as well as you how you are feeling. You know when you are tired or exhausted, hungry or thirsty, happy or unhappy, hopeful or despairing. No one knows as well as you what makes you leap for joy.

Only you will fully recall how you immersed yourself body and soul in a particular project or activity, and felt warmly, happily absorbed in it. You are the best expert on yourself, and you know best what does you good and enhances your health. While not a medical professional, you know what suits you, what strengthens you.

Are you ready not only to attend to the voice of your inner physician but also to act on what it is telling you?

Don't be discouraged if you can't yet answer this question with a clear 'yes'. Often life has carried us a long way away from dialogue with our inner physician or the habit of perceiving and feeling what we need. But we can learn to attend to this again.

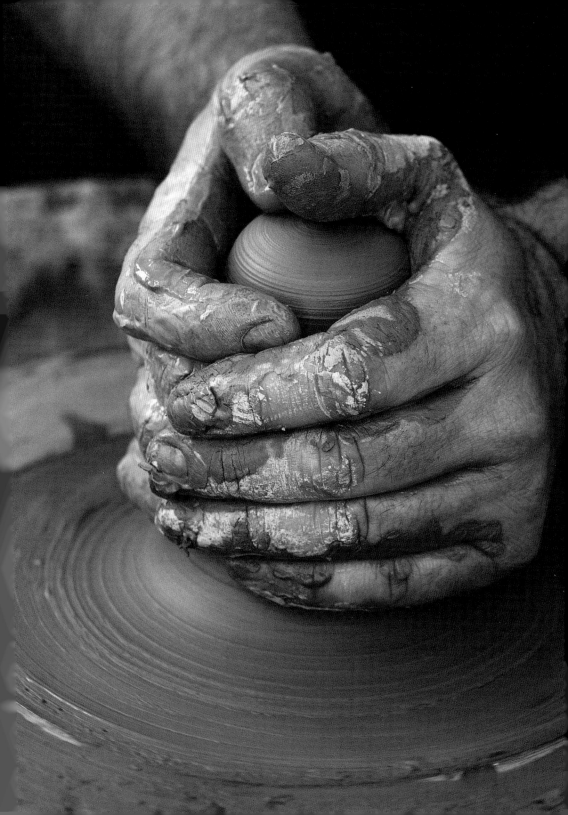

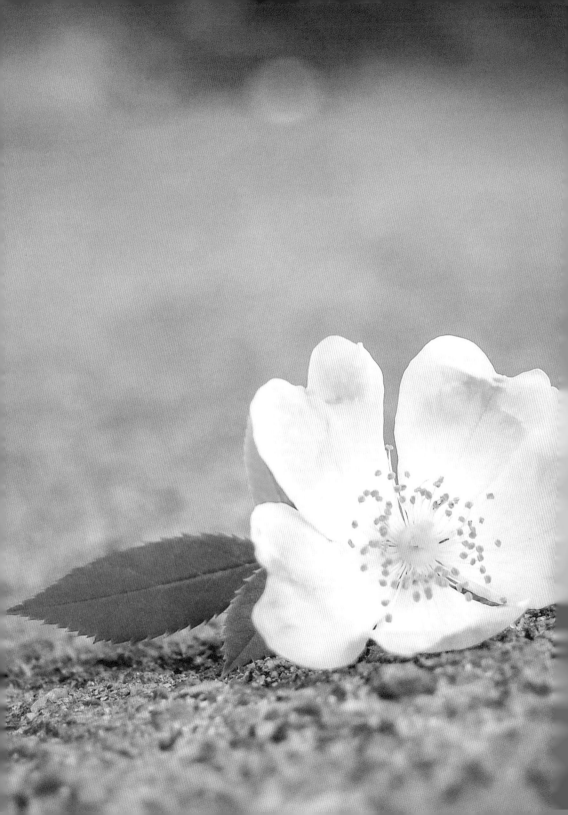

You Are

Your place is
where eyes regard you.
Where gazes meet
you come into being.

You are upheld by a call,
always the same voice:
it seems to be a single voice
with which all call.

You fell
but you are not falling now:
eyes sustain you.

You are
because eyes wish you to be:
they look on you and tell you
that you are.

Hilde Domin

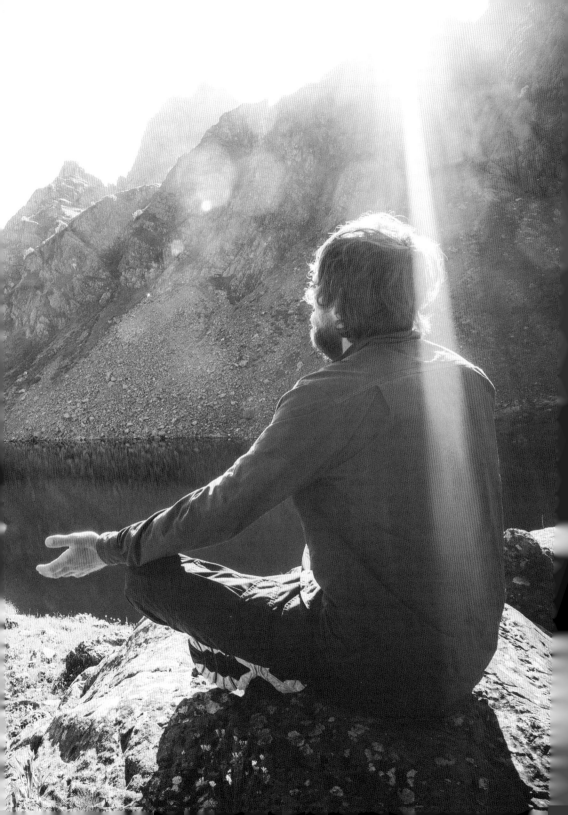

A Starting Point: our Threefold Relationship

You may be well and reading this book to stay well, or you may be ill and want to activate your self-healing forces to recover your health. Regardless, I'd like to start with a story that I think gives us insight into illness.

Re-tuning your instrument

In 1982 I worked in a Swiss clinic specialising in treating patients with cancer. One Sunday morning I happened to turn on the radio in my little office, and heard a broadcast sermon. It was a day of the year the Swiss call 'Day of the Sick' and so the minister was talking about disease.

He spoke about musicians having to regularly re-tune their instrument to be able to produce the right sounds, and he compared this with a period of illness. He said that while ill we have an opportunity to re-tune ourselves. Elaborating further, he described a threefold relationship in which each of us lives.

Each person, he said, has a relationship firstly with themselves, secondly with their fellow human beings and nature, and thirdly with the heavens, the universe and God. In this perspective, we exist in a three-way relationship.

The questions for each of us are: How am I living right now? Am I especially active in one of these relationships? To which do I give most attention? Are all three in balance?

The minister ended by summing up any period of illness as a time when we can rebalance the three relationships and thus re-tune our 'instrument'. Illness can be seen as a prompt to reconsider the balance and quality of each of these relationships in our lives.

An exercise: the threefold relationship in your life

Take a sheet of paper and sketch a diagram: a triangle of three equal sides, which takes up as much of the page as possible. Mark the middle of each side and draw lines to connect these mid-points. Now you have four small triangles inside the large one.

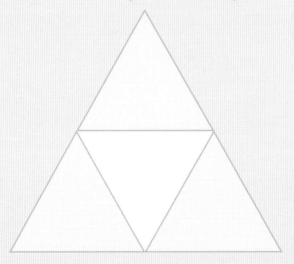

We will return to the triangles soon, but first take some time to think about how you feel right now in your relationship with yourself, with others and with the broader universe or God.

With yourself

❋ How is your relationship with yourself at the moment?

This question brings with it the task of perceiving your own needs – at all levels – and, where appropriate, stating them to the people around you. We need to acknowledge ourselves, to respect and value ourselves, as well as respecting and valuing others. And we need to recognise, respect and broaden our own limitations. For many of us, this can be the hardest of the threefold relationships to make time for. If it helps, consider marking out 'time for myself' in your diary or daily timetable.

With others

❋ How do you feel in your relationships with those closest to you: your family, friends and colleagues?

Does anything need to change here? How do you speak to each other? How well do you communicate with each other about what you experience, what you hope for and desire?

With the universe or God

❋ And how is your relationship to the heavens (or however you may like to think of this dimension)?

Have you been able to cultivate and maintain a religious or spiritual aspect to your life? Do you feel a vibrant enthusiasm? Do wonder, gratitude and stillness fill your days with joy?

Try to immerse yourself in your own sense of these three relationships in your life right now. How easy is it for you to engage with these questions?

We will return to your diagram and your sense of your threefold relationships shortly.

Over the past thirty years I have repeatedly encountered different variations of this threefold picture and I firmly believe it has many insights to offer us.

The connection with healing potential

Perhaps you can already sense how our quality of life in these three realms is intimately bound up with our potential for healing. As we recover from an illness, this threefold dialogue must be consciously cultivated. We need to open ourselves time and again to new experiences in these three relationships.

In which of the three fields would you begin a revived threefold conversation?

A dialogue with myself

Most people start with themselves.

Sometimes patients tell me that their way of life has plunged them into a sense of despair. They can no longer see a way forward and have lost all faith that they might improve their circumstances. Some even say that they no longer want to go on.

If you have felt similarly, perhaps this book can help you to experience things differently, to discover and develop your own potential, and to value it.

> Returning to the exercise, label the shape you drew, so that the three small triangles lying at the three angles of the large triangle say: 'with myself' in the first, 'with others' in the second and 'with God and/or the universe' in the third (if neither of these words has meaning for you, use your own word, or perhaps leave that third triangle empty for now). In the central small triangle, write the word 'I'. Then draw three arrows from the central 'I' triangle pointing to the other three triangles.
>
> Now give a colour to each of these three relationships in your own life.

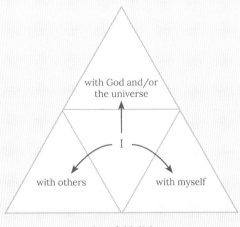

Our threefold dialogue

How do you experience these triangles? As the diagram stands, does it strike you as an accurate picture of your relationships, or do you feel that some change is needed to make it more genuinely reflective of your current situation? Should one of the triangles be smaller or another larger? How well connected should these triangles appear? Make the changes, so your diagram represents your threefold relationships as you experience them now.

Please draw a second diagram now. This one will show the way you *would like* your threefold relationships to feel. If you prefer, you can draw circles for this one instead of triangles. Give each segment a size and colour and connection to the central 'I'.

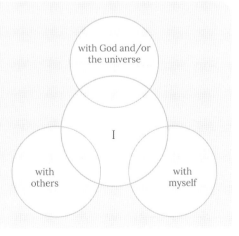

Once you have drawn the two versions of the diagram, consider how you might actually move from the first representation of how things are to the second, more harmonious picture. Note your thoughts, but for the time being keep this as an open question.

This book may provide ways of positively improving each of your threefold relationships. It may help you use a time of illness as a prompt to re-tune your instrument – to re-harmonise your life.

Keep your diagrams to return to on our journey towards

* understanding what nurtures your healing potential;
* finding a way to integrate these insights into your life, overcoming obstacles;
* and perhaps intuiting the meaning of the illness you have been suffering and the challenge it presents.

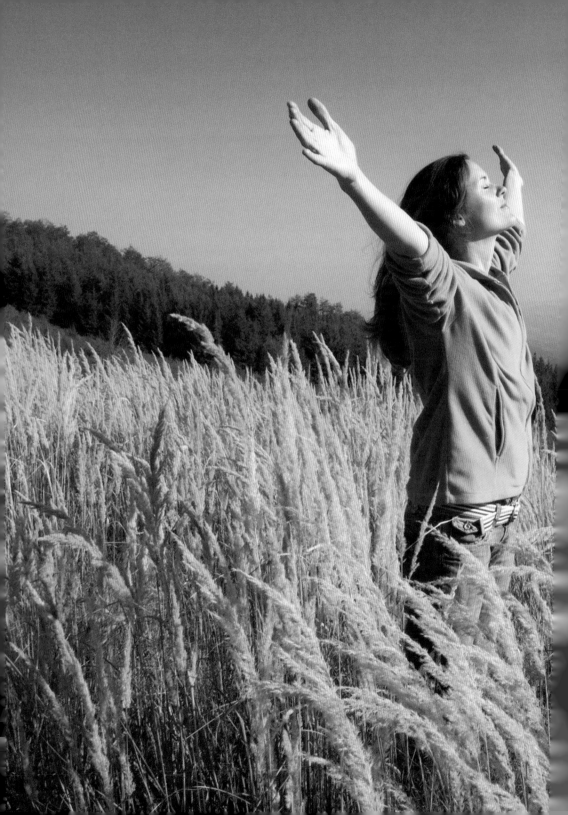

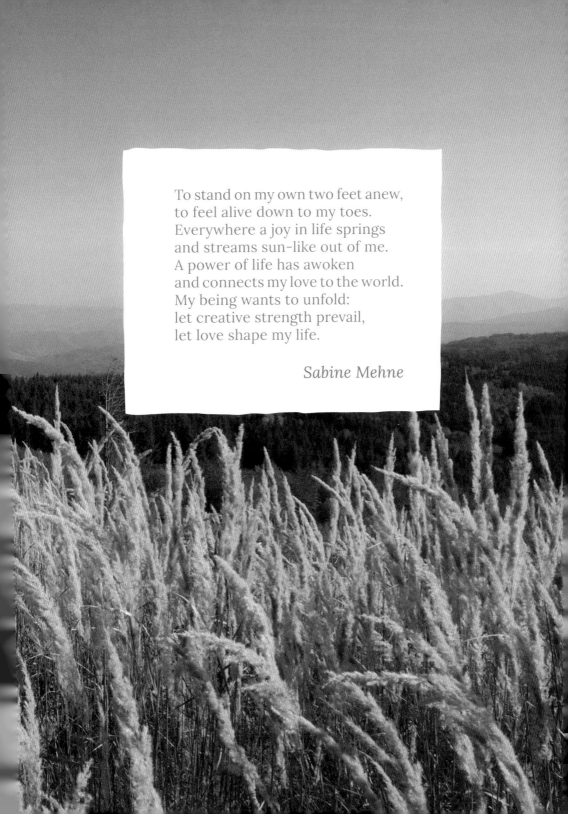

To stand on my own two feet anew,
to feel alive down to my toes.
Everywhere a joy in life springs
and streams sun-like out of me.
A power of life has awoken
and connects my love to the world.
My being wants to unfold:
let creative strength prevail,
let love shape my life.

Sabine Mehne

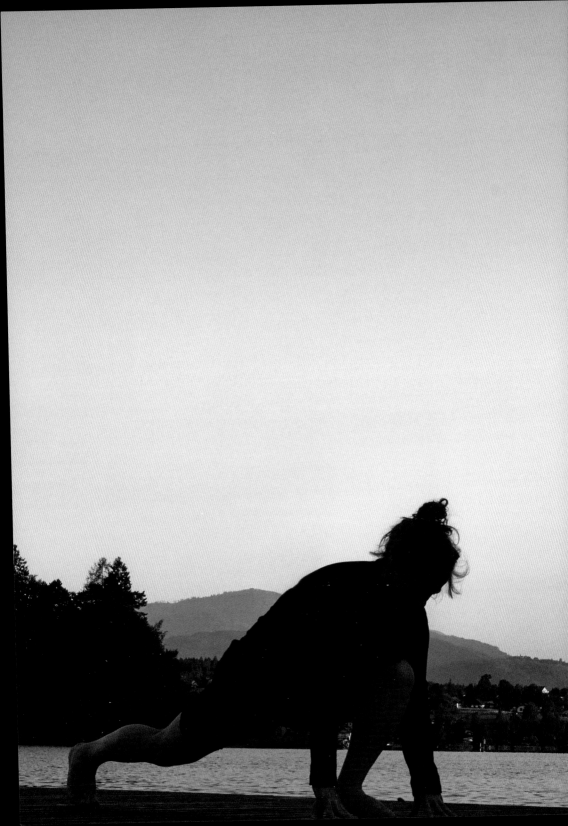

What is Health? Where Are We Travelling To?

In modern medicine, patients are urged to fight their illness. This often leads to them fixating on overcoming it at all costs. If this fails they give up hope. Instead, we would ideally be encouraged to accept our illness as an integral part of our biography, so that we learn not only to fight it, but also to live with it.

Don't be swallowed up by medicine

Medical ethicist Professor Giovanni Maio contrasts an increasingly technical medicine, driven by economic constraints, with a positive picture of patient care in which people learn to handle their own illness so that they don't feel completely swallowed up by the health system.

Often we think of ourselves as healthy only if we are in perfectly fit condition, but even those who are ill can be healthy if they learn to live with their illness in the right way. Being healthy means developing a creative relationship to your illness within the limits of your abilities; it is about our inner being.[6]

Consciousness and gratitude

In my work with people who have lived with illness for a long time, I often find that they are better able to cope with the realities of life than they were before they fell ill: they are more thankful and live more consciously. Awareness and gratitude are life-changing qualities to have gained on a journey through illness.

Everything we learn on our journey can help us cultivate 'inner health', enabling us to find meaning in illness and make peace with our situation. Such acceptance and new-found contentment has even been known to bring extra years of life to people who believed they were close to death.

Let us set off.

Facing a crisis such as an illness can be compared with a voyage of discovery to a new land, yet I suspect most of what you discover will be more like a memory of something you have always known.

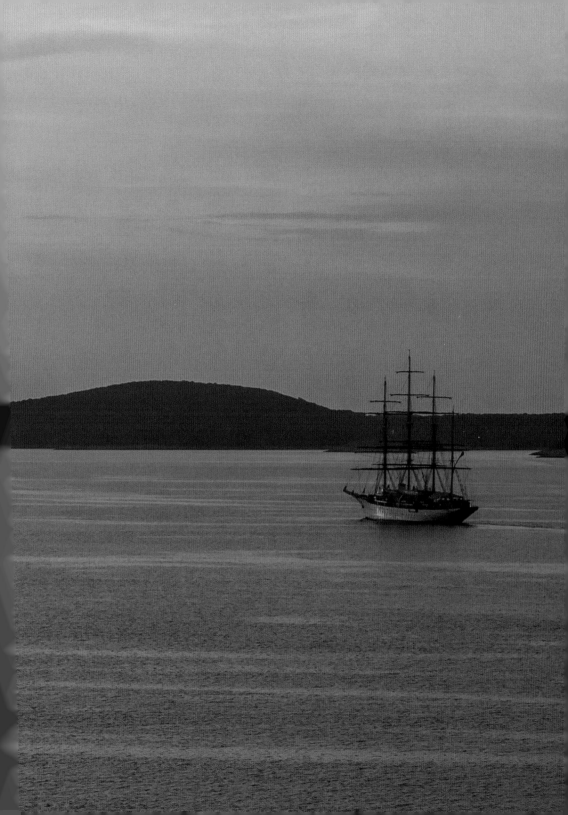

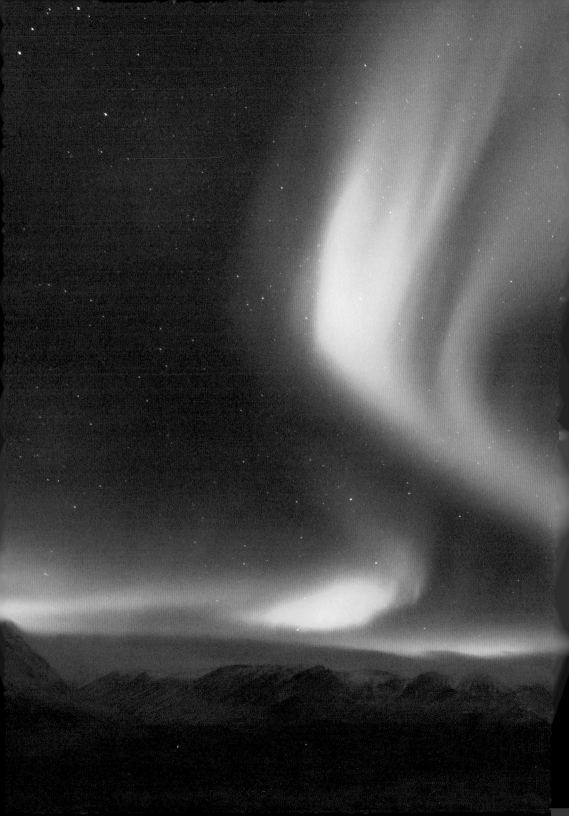

When we betray the truth
we betray ourselves.
It is not a question of lying
but of acting against one's conviction.

Novalis

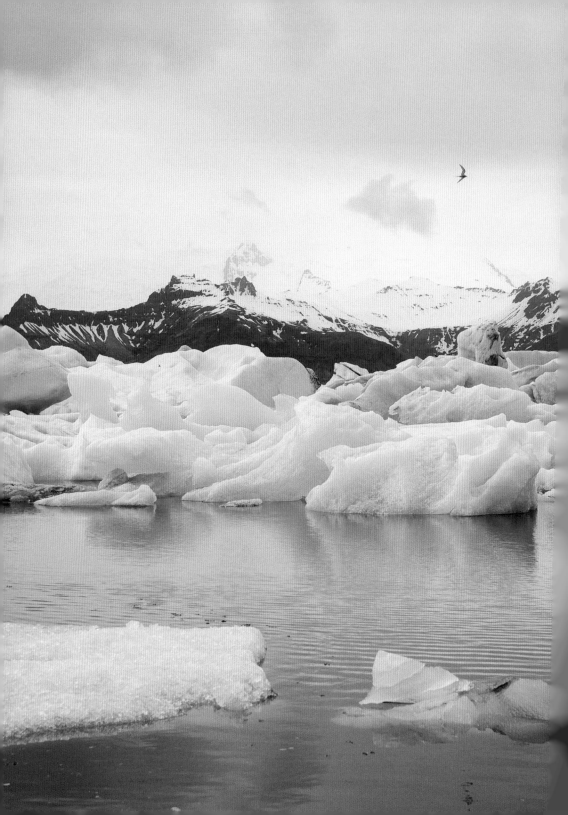

Prioritising Health: for the World, for the Individual

Can we conceive of 'humankind health', the health of us all? What kind of journey would we need to take before we could speak of humanity's health-giving influence on planet Earth? Whatever 'humankind health' might be, and however long the journey to humanity giving health to the Earth, each of us can only begin with our own thinking and actions. Can we make changes towards healing, for ourselves, for others, for the Earth?

People are increasingly aware of the need for a sustainable way of life that does not exploit and destroy the Earth any further. They increasingly question the dogma of perpetual growth. They long for a life in which the hope of a better future is no longer dismissed as a mere illusion.

There is a growing realisation that we really can shape our lives.

The paradox: illness and the good life

Outwardly it seems we in the West have never had it so good, and yet at the same time we have never been as 'sick' as we are now. Paradoxically our lifestyles produce systemic and chronic diseases such as diabetes and depression. We live in circumstances that make it ever harder to maintain a sense of our full humanity. It is ever harder to lead a self-determining life in which we accord full value to our own thinking, feeling and actions. This in itself leads to illness. Eventually our healthcare systems will collapse under the burden.

We live inside a materialistic ideology in which humans have become mere commodities: not only nature, but we too are being exploited. We are robbed of our humanity. If we go on prioritising economic efficiency and growth, profit maximization and exploitation of resources over human values, then damage to the Earth, to humanity and to our health will inevitably continue.

Give life priority

For things to change and heal we will have to prioritise the needs of life instead, whether natural or human. We need to take on a stance of nurturing the potential in all living creatures.

Society today often faces the same problems and issues that we face as individuals. The Earth and our society are in some ways 'sick', and change is needed to stimulate healing processes.

Many of us battle our way through the demands we encounter each day, our time and activity given up to external controls and compulsions, Are we even willing to heed what our body, our soul, our spirit is telling us?

Many people regard not only the world but their own body as a kind of object or machine rather than a living organism. To enhance its 'productivity' they exploit and medicate it. The results of such an outlook mount up.

Bodily limits

Many people push beyond the warning signs from their bodies. Some are dominated by the fear of loss; others desire to have still more; many are

A story: Paul's changing priorities

Paul is a brilliant computer scientist. His boss sent him all over the world, consulting with businesses and other researchers. His life was exciting and rewarding in many ways. It was also exhausting and depleting.

Now, suffering with an advanced tumour, he sits in front of me and says: 'I returned from an intense, three-week project in Canada. I was completely worn out. No sooner had I got home than my phone rang. It was my boss telling me to go to Bangkok the next day! I didn't say no. I didn't want to lose my job. Only now that I have cancer do I realise that I actually have a body and I am responsible for it. And only now do I realise what my priorities really are.'

Paul's difficult illness led him to change his priorities. Such crises offer us great learning and development potential.

unaware of what drives them to ignore their own limitations. Behaving as though we do not have bodies with absolute needs creates imbalances that are likely to lead eventually to crisis or illness.

It seems to me that many of us behave as though our bodies do not fully belong to us, or our children, or even the Earth itself. We have withdrawn from nature and ourselves and taken refuge in prescriptive rules, inherited systems of thought and received morality. In the world of work and our healthcare systems we have created such mechanised processes that our daily life is largely dictated by a cold and systematic functionality. Human concerns are lost within organisations that require fewer employees to carry out more tasks.

In his 2010 seminar 'Anxiety in the Modern World', the German neurobiologist Gerald Hüthner spoke of the increasing prevalence of 'self-suppression': the loss and destruction of the self.[7] According to a survey published in the magazine *Nature*, he said, around a third of the scientists questioned took psycho-stimulants to enhance their performance and to be able to work through the night. What kind of picture of the human being prevails here?

Creeping habituation

Two phenomena in animal research seem to offer some answers. The first is a gruesome experiment on live frogs: they are put in a saucepan of cold water and the water is slowly heated. Swimming in their accustomed element, the frogs do not recognise the threat as the temperature rises, but if another, 'unadapted' frog is placed in the saucepan, it immediately feels the heat and leaps out again. The others meanwhile, lulled into compliance, die without ever having recognised the danger.

In the second experiment, if you put fleas in a glass vessel with a lid, they keep knocking against it as they leap. But at some point they learn the constraints and no longer jump as high: they become conditioned. But if you then remove the lid and add new fleas, the newcomers adapt to the behaviour of the others and leap only as high as those already present, even though there is no lid holding them in.

Applied to human beings, the moral of the two stories is clear: we all too easily grow accustomed to the status quo or the conditioning imposed upon us from without. We often think we must comply with the systems imposed upon us and function within them as required.

I urge you to use your own perceptive faculties – your ability to know and feel – to find your own inner certainty and act accordingly.

Self-perception and inner knowledge

In coming to perceive and acknowledge ourselves, we become the best specialist in our own health. We can discover our own inner voice. I do not mean by this the conditioned dictates with which we have been indoctrinated, but a deeper knowing above and beyond society's teachings. I mean a certainty about what will enhance our own lives. We can stop and take time to perceive how we are feeling in body, soul and spirit.

Are you willing to perceive and affirm the deeper voice inside yourself?

Questions: am I being myself?

We continually face the question of our own authenticity.

* Am I giving truthful expression to who I am? Am I being myself? Or am I suppressing parts of myself in order to survive?
* Am I ready for a dialogue with myself?

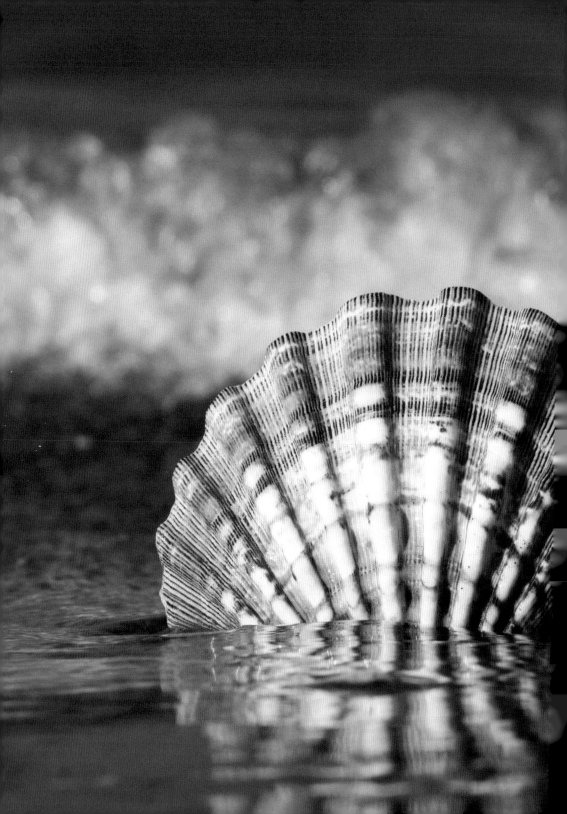

In yourself may God give you quiet pleasure,
an inward joy in his sweet flow of grace,
a sacred feeling that you belong together
with him, that in his eternal orders space
is made for you: a sense of uplift gained
by knowing yourself to be travelling the right
paths, and striving rightly for your aim.
Not self-importance, not risen to great height
and loftily looking down your nose at others,
but self-sufficient in your chosen way;
not arrogantly ploughing your own furrow
but honouring souls who share your destiny.
In self-content, at peace with all the world:
far from the busy tumult, close to God.

Friedrich Rückert

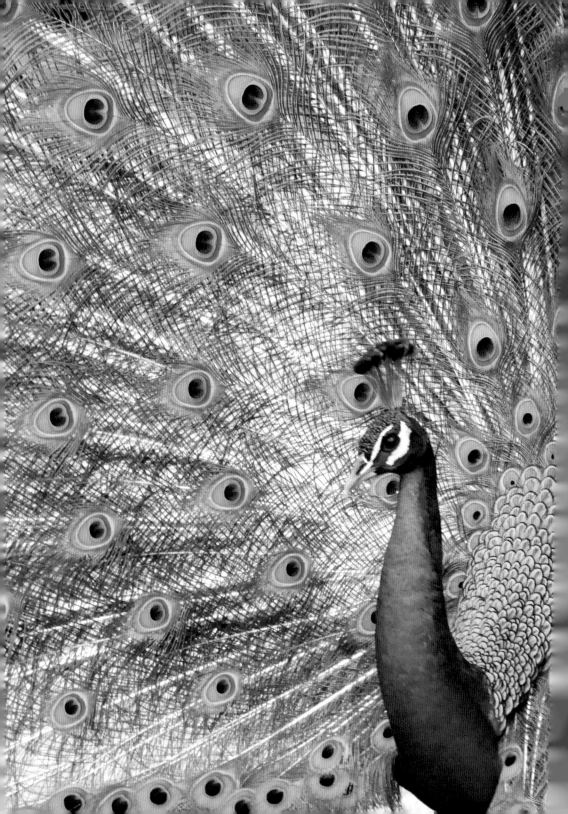

What Powers of Healing Lie Within?

Every illness is individual

Imagine a hundred patients with the same medical diagnosis: a tumour at exactly the same stage of progression. Imagine that each receives exactly the same form of treatment according to the latest medical standard. Will the outcome be the same for all of them? Almost everyone replies 'no' to this question. Of course not, they say.

What does this tell us?

Life shows that the same treatment can lead to very different results in different cases, although the patients apparently all have the same condition. The Canadian physician Sir William Osler (1849–1919), often regarded as the founder of modern medicine, once said: 'If it were not for the great variability among individuals, medicine might as well be a science and not an art.'[8]

I once had a group of health insurers and politicians visiting the therapy centre at our clinic, and I asked them why they thought the same treatment has such different results. Their spontaneous answer was that it was because people themselves are so different.

When I pursued this further and asked them in what way people were different, they cited two factors: outlook and constitution.

Each of us has our own nature, our own being. The differences between people, our individual mental, emotional and physical constitutions, are a very significant factor in illness and the process of recovery. We are *intrinsically* different from each other. Let us therefore examine more closely this primary element of variability in relation to healing.

My outlook has an effect

If, given our magnificent specialised medical knowledge, we focus exclusively on the biochemistry of the body, our minds can become filled to such an extent with this highly complex biochemical level of reality that we can lose sight of all other contexts. Beside measurable objective phenomena, it starts to seem unimportant how the body's present condition may have developed over time, and how this has been affected by inward and outward factors. The medical system diagnoses symptoms of illness, and decides these symptoms must be eradicated.

This can lead us to working only on tackling symptoms – which demonstrably does extend survival time and can enhance quality of life.

A sustainable cure

BUT if we seek an enduring, sustained process of healing that reaches deeper than the outward signs of illness – the symptoms – and tries to comprehend the underlying causes, we must concern ourselves also with the patient's individual circumstances. We must integrate real experiences or we run the risk of overlooking the patient's own life and outlook.

The context of treatment is also vital. We know from the placebo effect that the impact of the doctor–patient relationship is considerable.[9] The expectations of patients and doctors and the attitude of the doctor towards the medicine all have effects.[10]

Rather than surrendering to the technology of medicine, every person can actively affect their own health and can support their healing forces.

A story: Sara the physician

Sara, an internist, told me that in her work as a physician she gradually came to prescribe fewer and fewer medicines, instead giving more space during consultations to discussion with the patient. The medicines she did prescribe always had the desired effect. But when she took a three-month break from work in her practice and a replacement physician took her place, it became apparent that the medicines were no longer working adequately.

A patient later explained to her that the cover doctor handed out prescriptions with the words, 'Well, just continue with that then.' He didn't take time for discussion with patients. He didn't come across as respecting or believing in the treatment. And the medicine in itself was not enough.

A story: the power of the mind

In 1952, Dr Bruno Klopfer was studying a potential new cancer medicine, Krebiozen. The drug was tested on a number of patients, but only had a positive effect on one. This patient was extremely ill. He was confined to bed and was breathing through an oxygen mask. After treatment with Krebiozen, his condition dramatically improved. He was able to get up, and soon after that he left the clinic.

Because he had seen that the drug was ineffective on other patients, and because he had carefully observed the patient, Dr Klopfer was sure that this man's recovery was not the result of the medication but of his deep, inner conviction that the medicine would help him. Dr Klopfer wanted to prove this to his colleagues and so, after a while, he called the patient back to the clinic and offered him what he said was a still better, improved version of Krebiozen. In fact, he only administered a salt solution. He reported that the man's tumours melted away like snow balls on a stove.

Later, the clinical studies of Krebiozen were published. The drug was declared to be a failure and was not recommended for further use.

The patient who had been cured had continued to be interested in the drug, and he read the report. He returned to the clinic soon afterwards and died.

If it wasn't the Krebiozen, what was the power acting on the man's body and his tumours?[11]

A story: the power of visualisation

In 1971, US physician Dr Carl Simonton was treating a patient with radiotherapy. All his colleagues believed the case was hopeless. Dr Simonton asked the patient to try an experiment. He asked the man to spend five minutes each day visualising the treatment's success as vividly as possible.

The outcome of radiotherapy? A complete success. Still more astonishing was that the patient suffered no side effects.

Dr Simonton was so struck by the man's recovery, he began using visualisation in his treatment of every tumour patient.

It is worth noting that in 1971 the field of 'psycho-oncology' was still emerging – Dr Simonton was one of its pioneers – and none of the oncologists around Dr Simonton were interested in his new methods, indeed he was regarded with contempt for many years. There was a conviction that a patient's mental and emotional state bore no relationship to the biology of a tumour.

A question: self-fulfilling prophecy

Self-fulfilling prophecy means simply that a person carries in their mind, in their inner reality, a picture or idea that then becomes outward reality.

In your own life, have you felt or seen the effect of profound inner conviction?

The 'dual unity' of patient and illness

There is never only an illness, always a person and an illness. The person and the illness are a dual unity: they must be considered separately and together.

Sir William Osler taught his students:

> It is much more important to know what sort of patient has a disease than what sort of disease a patient has.

Just as the patient and illness are a dual unity, the patient's physical life and their soul or spiritual being are also a dual unity, to be considered both separately and together.

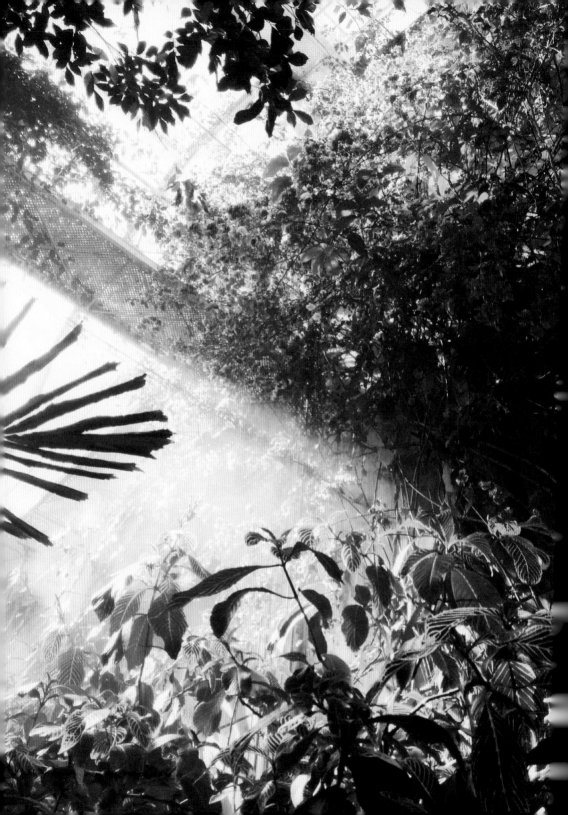

What helped to cure you?

Consider Caryle Hirshberg's 'cake graphs'. Hirshberg talked with people who had recovered from cancer, asking them about their experience and particularly what had helped them to recover. The patients reflected on all the positive influences on their recovery, then assigned each one a portion of a 'cake' depending on its significance.

Hirshberg collected thousands of these cake graphs. Each was unique, but in every one the slice given to 'medicine' was only a partial fraction of the cure.[12]

Questions: hearing the stories of others

❋ When you read or hear the stories of people who have recovered from severe illness, do you feel they can affect your own life and your own healing?

❋ Do the habits of thought we have all gained through science assist us in absorbing these stories and benefiting from them, or are they getting in the way?

A story: Geraldine – the power of joy and purpose

My patient Geraldine was diagnosed many years ago with a medically incurable tumour. She was expected to die in 2008, and then again in 2014. Very much alive, she sits in front of me full of the joy of life. After being declared incurable, she started working to help refugees in her home town. She shows me a picture on her phone of Niklas, a two-year-old refugee who wasn't coping with living in containers and became more and more unwell.

He was fostered by Geraldine and her husband. As she tells me about Niklas, she brims with joy and gratitude. In this purpose, she has found meaning in life and a sense of thankfulness, lovingly connected with a larger reality. She tells me that two weeks earlier she had a CT scan and her tumour remains in remission.

Make choices about your treatment

In a journey through illness, your inner state will be affected by your feelings about the treatment you're receiving: by whether or not you can affirm and accept it. Many patients say that they feel required to comply with what is prescribed for them. They speak as though they have landed in a system that processes them, as though they have lost their own power to decide. Many patients feel, 'Well, I will just have to go along with all this, get it over with, wait and see, perhaps I will recover.' They take on a mindset in which recovery is almost nothing to do with them.

Hopefully these patients will indeed recover. Yet if we acknowledge the power of the mind in our own health, we can see that our own deeply help beliefs about whether our treatment will help us or harm us must make a significant difference to the outcome.

Healthy activities in your days

People who sing in a choir or who become immersed in a creative artistic project know the enlivening effect such activities can have. You can feel them doing you good: body, mind and soul.

Questions: staying in touch with yourself

Whether you are dealing with severe illness or are in good health, take the time to look inward every now and then. Ask yourself:

❋ How am I?
❋ What is the direction of my thoughts and feelings?
❋ Are they in line with my actions?
❋ How am I shaping things for myself?
❋ How active am I in what is happening in my own life?

Healthy people in your life

Physician and psychotherapist Dr Wolf Büntig came to the end of a lecture on cancer and said, 'I can give you one piece of simple, firm, absolute advice.' There was a sense of expectancy in the room as the audience waited. He said:

> Surround yourself with healthy people; health is infectious!
> Healthy people are those with whom you can laugh and cry; those whom you can hug.

Laughter is healing

In laughter and play the soul liberates itself from the body's chains and breathes more freely. And with the liberation of the soul, the body too breathes deeper. New life energy streams through it. Research has found that white blood corpuscles form when we laugh, sustaining our immune system. Indeed there is some evidence that heartfelt laughter triggers the formation of more white blood corpuscles than any other emotional state. Laughter stimulates circulation, enhances digestion and much more.[13]

63

An exercise: what gives you pleasure? What gives your life meaning?

Ask yourself the following questions:

* When do I feel inspired and enthusiastic?
* What strengthens and energises me?
* Which people make me feel particularly well? Sometimes we find that being with certain people takes a lot of our energy. Is there anyone in your life like this?
* Can you recall days when you have felt joy and gratitude? What happened on those days? What were you doing? Who were you with?

Consider all your answers and list the people and activities that give you great pleasure and enthusiasm. List what brings you a sense of meaning and fulfilment.

The influence of our thoughts

It is normal to feel both hope and despair. But notice if you are becoming stuck in hopelessness. Seek help and support to emerge from it again.

Our thoughts can enhance or inhibit the release of our physical resources. It is important to ask how our feelings arise and to consider positive ways of dealing with them. Most of us are not taught how to recognise and work with our own emotions. Try to notice what gives rise to your own hope or despair, especially in connection with illness, with treatment, even when life is ending. Do the ideas, pictures and stories in your head reinforce hope, courage and trust? Could they?

Exercises: is there another way to see this?

Try these exercises when you are anxious, or find that the same thoughts are revolving around and around your head.

When we are stuck in 'hamster-wheel thinking' negative thoughts seem to imprison us. This can lead to us feeling extremely unwell. Such thoughts can paralyse and block us, and can be so insistent that we can think of nothing else.

Imagine a ball that has a different colour on each quarter. From where we are standing, we see a blue ball. The person opposite us sees a red ball. But we are both looking at the same object. Although we are both looking at the same ball, we will only see what the other person sees if we let go of our own angle of vision and move to stand where they stand.

Similarly, when we are stuck in the hamster wheel, our perspective is often restricted, and so insistent that it seems the only possible way to see life. When people are stuck like this, it is not surprising that they may distract themselves with compulsive activities or use substances that numb their awareness.

* The first step is to recognise that we are stuck in compulsive thoughts. This will immediately give us a little bit of distance.
* Second, sit down and simply observe the thoughts that come.
* Then take the time to write them down. This will help us detach from the fixed position of the victim.
* Look at the thoughts written down. How closely do these ideas connect to reality? Ask someone you trust to tell you what they think too. Do your compulsive thoughts represent a full picture of reality?

When we are facing times of psychological distress, our thoughts tend to arise from our subconscious, from fears and doubts, rather than from dispassionate observation and a broad view of the facts.

Once we have recognised our habitual thoughts and written them down outside of ourselves, we are in a position to question them, to change them. But it is is also true that letting go of accustomed thoughts is one of the most difficult challenges we all face.

As you read through this book, there will be more ideas to help you with this challenge.

Accepting negative thoughts

The knowledge that our mind can exert a positive influence and impact on organic processes in our body creates a sense of pressure for many people. They feel an unhappy responsibility for their thoughts and for their illness, and believe they should never feel sad, or entertain negative thoughts, that they *must* think positively! Yet this simply exchanges one inner compulsion for another.

Instead, we can see what is solved with time and patience. It is important to feel what lives within us, including sadness and rage. All our emotions need to be perceived, acknowledged and accepted, including the negative ones. As we make our way through fear or grief, something transforms in us, matures, strengthens.

I believe that it is harder to cope with life if we are always intent on what should or should not be. A gentler way is to acknowledge what is and affirm it.

Despair and hope

Despair says, 'Nothing is any use, I won't get better. I will lose everything. I can't do anything, I'm a failure.'

Hope says, 'Help is always possible. However ill I am, life can always bring healing.' Even (and this may sound strange or contradictory), 'I can find healing before I die.'

Fear and trust

What would we discover if we studied situations in which some people feel fear and others don't? What is different about those who are not anxious, despite, say, having a grave illness or an uncertain future hanging over them? There are people who went to their execution, their death, with relative tranquillity – Socrates, Hans and Sophie Scholl, Dietrich Bonhoeffer. What was different about these people compared to many of us?

What kind of trust lives in people like that?

I was struck by the words of one of my patients, who had a serious illness yet an inner steadiness. She said with conviction, 'Whatever happens, things will end well for me!'

Strengthening immunity and beyond

In modern tumour science, increasing attention is being given to the tumour's micro-environment, to the way its immediate cellular environment influences its development. A tumour's surrounding cells

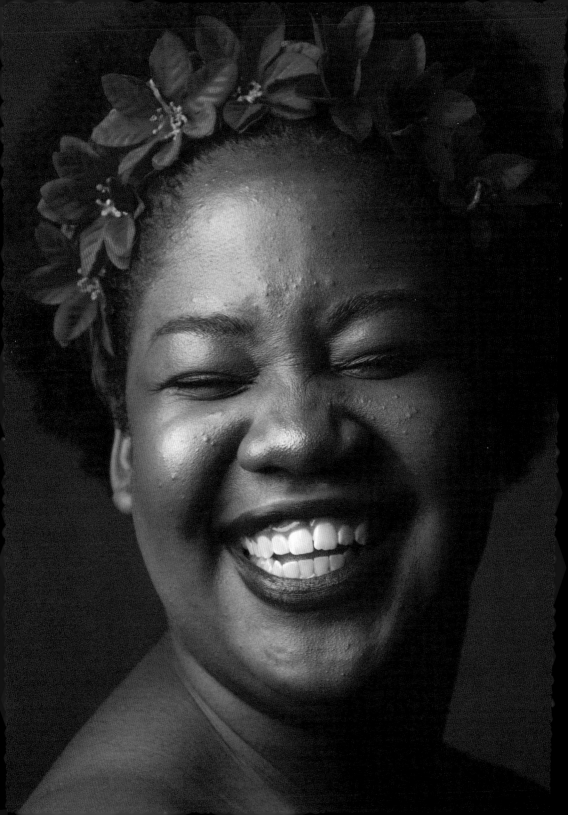

make a great difference to its progress. Our bodies' healthy organising forces can suddenly get a grip on what is happening or they can be blocked from intervening.

Strengthening the immune system so that it can engage with the tumour cells is a very different medical approach to externally attacking and combatting the tumour. Cancer immune therapy has now become a firmly established part of mainstream treatment.

Even when we are helped by medical breakthroughs like immune therapy, there is still room for recognising the healing potential in a patient's soul and spirit. Once psycho-immunology was dismissed; now a patient's psychology is seen as central to their treatment. Perhaps in the long term we can look forward to the whole person, including the spiritual person, being reintegrated into medical procedures.

A force for constant repair

Let us consider the defensive forces within our bodies. The medical journalist Kurt Langbein documented his own experience with cancer in the film *Miracle of Healing*. He said in an interview:

> For me, healing means re-establishing lost balance in the human system. It is very clear from modern neurobiology that body and mind are an indivisible unity. When this unity is in balance, it can cope with many health challenges, including the 10,000 to 100,000 cancer cells that develop each day in every one of us. We all get this cancer all the time as normally occurring cell division failure.[14]

The daily process of tumour-cell eradication within us can be disrupted. When this happens we need to remedy the disturbance and strengthen the forces of healthy, healing bodily re-organisation. This cannot happen at the flick of a switch; it requires time and attention, insight, resolve and the capacity to act. Even if we do make all these efforts there is no guarantee we will achieve the desired outcome. Yet still it makes sense to embark on this path.

Wounds, scabs and the process of healing

We have all watched wounds heal, and may not even have thought much about it. When our skin is injured, our bodies create a protective layer over the wound, a scab. Scabs look damaged and messy, but they are there for a reason. Scabs are much tougher and more resilient than skin. They are a tough crust that allows the wound to heal underneath.

Imagine if we did not know that scabs are protective. Imagine if we didn't understand that the scab was just one stage in healing, that it was temporary. If we didn't understand scabs, we might regard one as being in itself the problem: something we must eradicate, a pathological condition.

Is it possible that this mistaken attitude to scabs is in fact the kind of attitude we take to serious illness? We call a set of symptoms 'sick' because we cannot see the whole process. We do not wait to see what happens to the whole organism over time; we do not predict what the illness makes possible.

When does illness begin?

As our diagnostic technologies develop, it will become increasingly possible to detect small cellular disturbances at an ever-earlier stage. The question of when we actually become ill will be ever more in question.

Will we – do we even now – intervene in 'illnesses' that would have been resolved by the body without medical intervention?

Did you know that your body has entirely renewed itself several times during your lifetime? It does so roughly every seven years. *The part of your body that is sick at present has repeatedly reorganised itself healthily and wholesomely up to the time when you became ill.*

When we think about the body's capacity for renewal and repair, consider the lungs. If we take two x-rays of a smoker's lungs, the first the day she quits for good and the second two years later, we will see that during those two years the lungs will have renewed themselves. The tar will have disappeared.[15]

Without you thinking about it, the temple of your body is constantly being rebuilt. Every day an unimaginable miracle is occurring within you.

The body's organising wisdom

We do not have a name for the forces that organise and invigorate the body – we tend to take them for granted until they do not work. We could think of them as the powers of the universe, or of the heavens. Some doctors speak of a 'blueprint', a kind of archetype always present in the body.

If we could consciously observe the processes of building, repairing and transforming that our body accomplishes all the time, we would develop a great deal of trust in this organising wisdom at the biochemical level. Every day, though we are unaware of it, a process of complete dissolution and destruction of the food we eat takes place in our metabolism. Our body breaks down foreign substances completely, then synthesises its own substances from them. Our bodies need to be able to break down other forms of matter to create themselves and develop their own individual lives. We embody a kind of courage in chaos.

But what wisdom of futurity chooses and reconfigures particular cells from this endless, chaotic potential? What power decides which of the many developmental possibilities will be taken up? How does our coherent body renew itself from such chaos?

An exercise: considering the organising force in your own body

We have cells in our body that are an expression of illness. These cells have a dynamic of their own, they are in a sense autonomous: they do not take up the formative and differentiating impulses which cells in this place in the body took up before. Healthy cells, on the other hand, acquire a quite specific form and configuration that is appropriate for their place in the body.

The 'sick' cells were healthily configured before they became dysfunctional. Like all other healthy cells, they were pervaded by a formative organising force.

Think about what name you would give to the formative organising force in your own body that is even now keeping almost all your cells healthy and helping them form in the right way.

❋ Do you think of this as a spiritual or material force? Or both? Is it inside you, outside you, around you?
❋ Where was this force – which for decades maintained a healthy balance in your body between breakdown and build-up – when you become ill? What was happening for this force at that time?
❋ Do you feel that the force organising transformation and renewal, guiding the breaking down and building up of your cells in your body, has disappeared entirely?

Write your answers down.

Death and renewal

Without continual death in our organism, no renewal could occur. We need the capacity of death in order to live, in order to maintain the health of our organism.

All these processes, which are quietly accomplished by the wisdom active in our organism, are beyond the reach or governance of our conscious mind. Each day, in a sense, our organism passes through death and rebirth, and without this capacity it could not survive. In an adult human body, approximately five million cells die every second, and are renewed.[16]

Healthy reconfiguration

Healing only happens when our bodies' organising force, our power of healthy reconfiguration, returns to its natural scope. To put it very simply: healing happens when health once again permeates the place where the illness currently resides.

The most common and widespread medical treatment is oriented primarily to combating a lack or deficit. But to achieve a lasting cure, it is good to broaden our perspective beyond this narrow view of illness. It is good to embark on a journey that leads us not only to external 'specialists' but also to our own inner 'universalist'.

Positive and negative emotions are part of life. The decisive question is how much space and time they take up? Long-lasting despair, worry, anxiety, rage, hatred or grief weaken the immune system. Find help and support to create an outer and inner life in which there is joy and gratitude, and in which you feel you are shaping your own destiny.

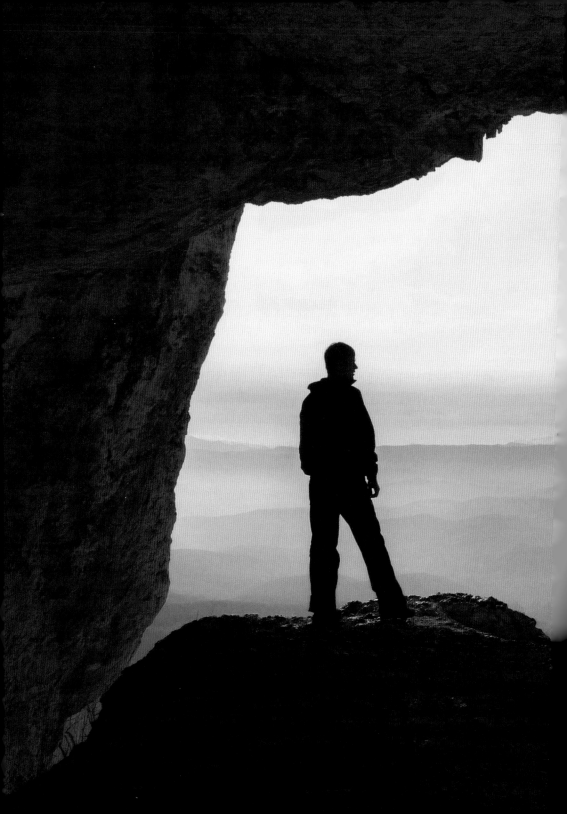

What happens when people open their hearts?

They get better.

Haruki Murakami

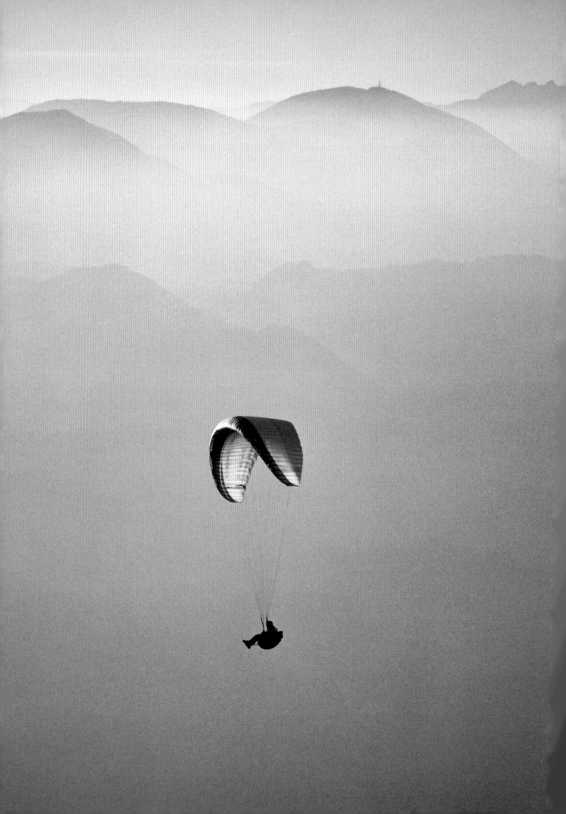

We Already Know How to Heal

Here is a hopeful thought. I believe that each of us bears within ourselves an awareness of what we need, of what is right for us, of our individual purpose on this Earth. This awareness has links to our conscience, our deep-seated knowledge of what is right and just. This awareness has not been taught to us, it does not come from parents or grandparents, it is not dominated by cultural norms, but is rooted in our true nature. Each person can find this awareness inside themselves, though it may take a long and difficult search. If we do search, a moment can come when an inextinguishable light of clarity and self-guidance emerges in the darkness.

People are more or less developed in their awareness of what they personally need, of what helps them thrive as an individual. But we all have the potential to develop this awareness further, to move towards health. We all also have the potential of course to ignore awareness and to move towards illness – this tendency is apparent around us every day. The clarity within us about what we need for our health, what is our purpose and what is good and just and right can be lost in times of trauma and extreme stress. We become rigid, follow agendas that are not our own, become stuck in patterns that are not helpful for us. It can take the shock of illness to start listening inwardly again and make radical changes in our own lives.

Does an awareness of what you need seem an abstract and unfounded idea to you? Nevertheless, I invite you to embrace it, at least as a possibility, and to persist with what might initially seem unfamiliar or strange.

Illness can lead to life-enhancing change

Rather than lamenting the problems we all face in the world, I believe there are more and more people resolved to engage and change things. They find a strength in themselves that carries them beyond fixed modes of thinking and behaving.

Crisis and illness can, paradoxically, act as a wellspring of energy in this respect. Each of us has within us an awareness of what we need, and also the capacity to change conditions for ourselves, and for the world more broadly. We can all move towards life-enhancing change. Illness may be part of what leads us to this change. We need to follow the path of belief, will, trust and love.

Patient autonomy in health care

Just as in the contemporary world we increasingly insist upon transparency in the political world and freedom of information, more and more patients in the health-care system want to understand their treatment and participate in decisions about their treatment. Medicine is becoming increasingly technical and yet top-down decisions are no longer appropriate. Health professionals may struggle with giving patients autonomy, as autonomy is hard to fit into a system. But without it, relationships become functional, rather than genuine encounters that contain the possibility of transformation.

The big question is whether there is still scope within a particular health system for real therapeutic or curative processes to unfold. No matter which treatment regime is employed, it is a central part of the curative relationship that both the patient and the healthcare worker are human beings with an inalienable dignity. Health is inevitably a less likely outcome if the system degrades both or either of them into mere objects.

The atmosphere in a hospital is a decisive factor in the success of treatment. Yet underfunded health care regularly leads to long waiting times for patients, to low staff morale, and to stress for all.

Above all else, patients need to be acknowledged as human beings. Patients need respect, they need to be regarded as competent – indeed to be regarded as the expert in their own health. Care that can see the full human being is more likely to lead to lasting health improvement rather than a quick-fix suppression of symptoms. The competent patient learns discernment in this field – and we are all potentially competent!

A picture of the future

To follow our path to recovery, we need a vivid picture of the future we want and need, and the knowledge that we can realise it.

Healing is possible

Hold this truth in mind: at a cellular level the body is constantly doing its own healing as we go about our lives, without any medical intervention.

Exercises: healthy cell regeneration

Imagine normal healthy cells at a particular place in the body. In the usual course of things most of these cells die and are renewed. Depending on the type of cell, their life span can be very different: days, weeks, months or years. Some cells last a whole lifetime.

I'd like to suggest a simple image to help us think about new cell formation. If you wish to, you can replace this image later with one you create yourself, but first try my suggestion:

* Open your hand wide, spreading out the fingers. Let's use this open hand as our image of a healthy developed cell, full of life.
* Now form your hand into a small ball. This fist can be our image of an embryonic stem cell.
* Slowly open your hand. This is our image of a healthy cell developing. Gradually unfold your hand and extend the fingers, spreading them out. This is an image of a cell's healthy development.
* Repeat this developmental process from the fist to the outstretched hand several times very slowly, feeling and experiencing it fully. To start with keep your eyes open as you do so, but then shut them and feel the process more inwardly. Think about the process of healthy cell formation occurring throughout your body – millions of cells are indeed developing in your body while you do this exercise.

Sometimes a cell does not extend fully, but stops mid-development.

* To picture this, half unfold your fist, then stop.
* Now take your other hand and help your half-opened hand extend completely.

When our organism is healthy, a continual dialogue occurs within and between cells. Cells help themselves and each other to develop fully. Just as a kind of dialogue of developmental support can arise between your hands, so cells support each other to grow and function healthily.

Cells also help each other repair when they become injured. The body is continually healing itself.

* As a picture of a healthy cell being injured, start with your hand fully spread, then curl your fingers inward.
* Use the other hand to help extend the fingers again. This is an image of the cell healing.

Illness from disrupted or damaged cells

Malignancy can arise from a halt in cellular development, from disturbed cell division or from cell damage. One type of tumour is caused by the failure of stem cells to develop into the specific configuration required at its location in the organism. These cells remain at an embryonic stage. This happens in some forms of leukaemia.

Malignancy can also develop in cells that have already formed healthily. In every cell, the DNA is injured continually and is healed again. If this normal ongoing healing process is disrupted, malignant cells may form.

A damaged cell's healthy form can be recreated anew in processes of dialogue within and between cells, but where these processes are disrupted, malignancy may develop. This can be the case with breast or colon cancer and other carcinoma types.

The following quote can help us understand the almost unimaginable work of DNA repair going on in our bodies all the time:

Considering causes of disorders in the genetic matrix, we think primarily of external influences such as radiation, chemical toxins or viruses. In fact, a considerable proportion of DNA damage arises from normal intracellular processes that are integral to our life and which are beyond our sphere of influence: failings in DNA synthesis (replication), spontaneous deamination of nucleotides or the forming of aggressive compounds such as oxygen radicals in the context of energy release, which damage inherited information in the cell nucleus and the mitochondria.

Whenever a cell divides, tens of thousands of mutations occur. If we consider that each human being is composed of 10^{14} cells, it is easy to understand that the risk of mutation is constant and extremely high. Yet most humans live for many decades. We owe our life expectancy to a series of highly effective defence systems.

Our bodies have built-in DNA repair systems that recognise very diverse types of cell error and eradicate them with enormous precision. After replication of the three billion base pairs in every cell, only around three errors remain in each cell. For comparison, imagine typing a million pages of text at 3,000 characters per page in only a few hours, and making no more than three typing errors. This is how thorough the DNA repair systems are in your body, and they have been at work maintaining your cells every day of your life.[17]

If we are ill, then these repair systems have been disrupted or blocked. But it is always possible that this disruption or block might be remedied, and the organising force that works in the body could begin to do its work again, as before.

Thus, in a simplified and metaphorical way we could say that illness arises due to a disruption of inter- and intracellular dialogue. But this doesn't mean that the disturbance cannot be recognised and remedied. The potential for our cells to remedy disturbance exists inside all of us; it has always been there.

Continuous becoming

Evolutionary biologist Wolfgang Schad founded his research on the principle that all life is constantly developing and evolving.

> No organism is static; each one is continuously active. There is no cell in our body in which breakdown and synthesis do not continually occur. ... Everything is always in a state of becoming rather than fixed existence.

> The world is always evolving, and once we know this we have a great aid in understanding ourselves. In trying to specify what the human being is we have to acknowledge that we are more than can be described. Why? Because we always have the potency or the quality to become something other than we have so far been. ... The human being only exists in as far as it is developing. This is a linguistic paradox. But if we recognise this and its significance for our understanding of ourselves and the world, we open up enormous potential for our development into the future.[18]

Who do doctors usually see?

Compare the likely mindset of a doctor who always works with patients who recover, to a doctor who works with the dying. When anyone experiences a sequence of events repeatedly, they will start to see it as expected, as perhaps inevitable.

Now consider that hospitals are, of course, dominated by patients whose condition is bad or has deteriorated. Patients who improve or recover no longer need to attend hospitals or consult doctors, or nowhere near so much. So medical practitioners are exposed predominantly to cases where illness is getting worse.

It is easy for those working in acute and palliative care wards to lose sight of the fact that they only have one particular perspective on a whole spectrum of reality. It is natural that their experience colours their view and leads them to be very wary of any hope of positive improvements in their patients, let alone recovery.

Of course it is important to be well prepared for the end of one's life, yet at the same time we must maintain hope in possibilities that seem miraculous and inexplicable: in improvement that comes not from without, through medical intervention, but from within, through the unfolding potential of life. Experience has shown that such turnarounds are a reality, and we should remember this.

Miracles

It is unrealistic not to believe in miracles.

Walter M. Gallmeier [19]

The power of the spirit

The great German Enlightenment writer and thinker Friedrich Schiller said, 'It is the spirit which builds the body.' He lived much of his life in fragile health, but was sustained, and spurred into impressive productivity, by his belief that the spirit was primary, and could accomplish much, regardless of the state of the body, indeed that the life of the spirit would benefit the body. Schiller was gravely ill with tuberculosis before he died, but he continued to write and to be active. After his death, the doctor conducting the post-mortem was astonished that he could have survived so long, and that he achieved so much in his last months.[20]

A story: powerful thoughts

A doctor told me the story of his patient, a young man who was suicidal after conflict with his partner. The doctor provided him with what he said were anti-depressant tablets, but the young man used them in massive overdose and was taken to hospital. Emergency ward staff tried to stabilise his condition, but he worsened and they declared him to be in danger of death.

The hospital staff made contact with the young man's doctor to enquire about the medication he had been prescribed. The doctor went to the ward immediately and explained to the young man that the pills he'd taken to poison himself were part of a research study and were placebos. They couldn't kill him.

The life-threatening symptoms disappeared, and shortly afterwards the young man felt so well again he was able to walk out of the clinic unaided, to seek, we hope, further help with his depression.

This story shows the power of our thoughts, of our mental pictures. We can literally think ourselves fatally unwell. Our beliefs can bring into being a physical reality.

Do you believe that if we can think ourselves fatally unwell with massive effect, we can also think ourselves healthier?

Positive thinking affects minds and bodies

It is a well-known fact in education that pupils develop differently depending on the teacher's attitude to them. The belief and trust of others, and of course our own trust in ourselves, have an effect: they help us realise our potential.

People who tend to think positively cope better with illness. People who say they are happy have stronger immune systems than those who report feeling unhappy. How much control, though, do we have over our feelings of happiness or unhappiness?

What we know we can control are the thoughts and experiences we cultivate. Each of us decides what we read, what we listen to, what we take an interest in.

Hope

When he was aged around 100, the philosopher Hans-Georg Gadamer (1900–2002) stated that much had changed in the field of philosophy during his lifetime but that one thing had remained the same: a human life was not possible without hope.

Illness as 'creativity-deficiency syndrome'

Our ideas of what we can or cannot do either constrain us or open up new horizons. At a time of crisis, of illness, we can form new ideas and thoughts, and extend our own limits.

Creativity can have a major role in change and recovery, yet often we fail to acknowledge our creative abilities. Creativity is a power we can draw upon, indeed, I believe that illness might be seen as an expression of 'creativity-deficiency syndrome'. Cure, it seems to me, is closely connected with accessing the creative powers within us. This in turn relates to capacities of wonder, thankfulness, courage, trust and, especially, the ability to love oneself.

86

Faith

In times of illness we feel our own lack of control – there are many events in our own lives that we do not choose. It can help to relinquish control, to hand yourself or your fate to a higher force. A cancer patient told me that the oncology professor in charge of her case said: 'This chemotherapy I am giving you is only a third of your treatment. Another third lies with you, and the last third is in the hands of God.' She found this comforting, and she trusted the professor.

Questions: faith

Those who can open themselves to a divine world draw inestimable help and strength from their belief. Many people who are cured of serious illness attribute their recovery to the power of prayer and faith.

Many others do not believe in a 'power beyond'.

❋ What does your own inner voice say?
  Faith and prayer involve acknowledging that we are not alone, and that we can find support and succour even in the direst need. For many people, faith and prayer bring trust and inner peace amid doubt.

❋ Can you recall any times in your life when you did not know how to go on, followed by moments when you felt surrounded and pervaded by a strength and wisdom which helped you?

Meaning

Hope is not optimism, nor the conviction that something will end well, but the certainty that something has meaning whatever the outcome.

Václav Havel

A story: Reinhold and the yellow rose

In 1987, Reinhold, a good friend of mine, lay in hospital close to death. He told his beloved partner that I would be coming and would bring him a yellow rose. This was a strange thing to say, as we hadn't spoken, he hadn't asked me to visit him or mentioned anything about a yellow rose, nor was I in the habit of bringing friends roses.

On the morning of St John's Day, one of my patients, nicknamed Iron Gustav, and a wonderful rose grower, visited me in the art therapy studio and, for the first time in all the years we had known each other, he brought me a rose. That morning, as he walked round his garden, he had been especially charmed by a rose with heavenly fragrance, a yellow rose, which he picked and brought for me.

Toward midday I got news that Reinhold had died the night before and was laid out. I wanted to visit him. It was immediately clear to me that I could bring him nothing more beautiful than the yellow rose I had received from Iron Gustav.

When I walked in, carrying the rose, his partner was amazed, as was I when she told me of Reinhold's words.

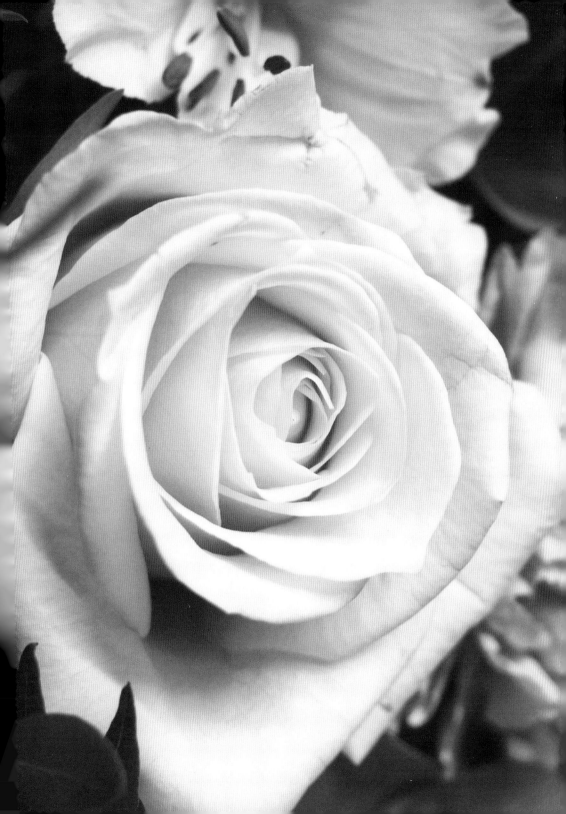

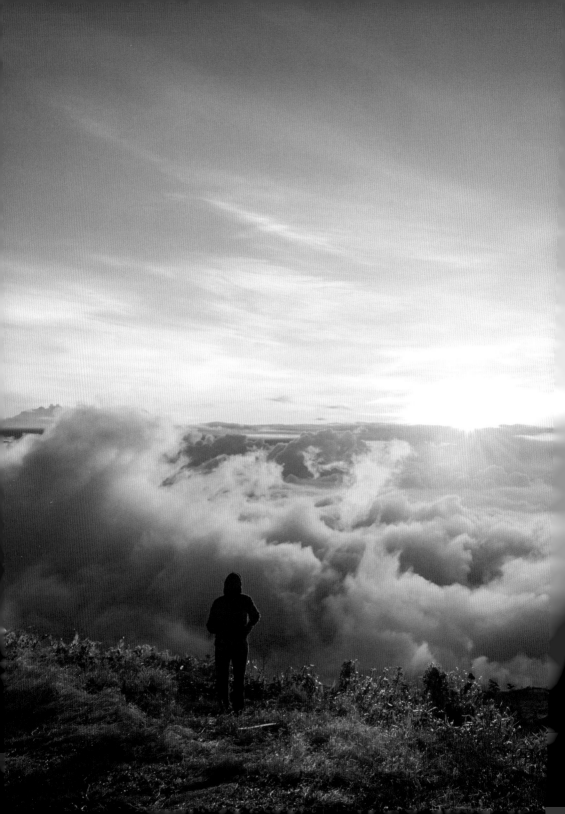

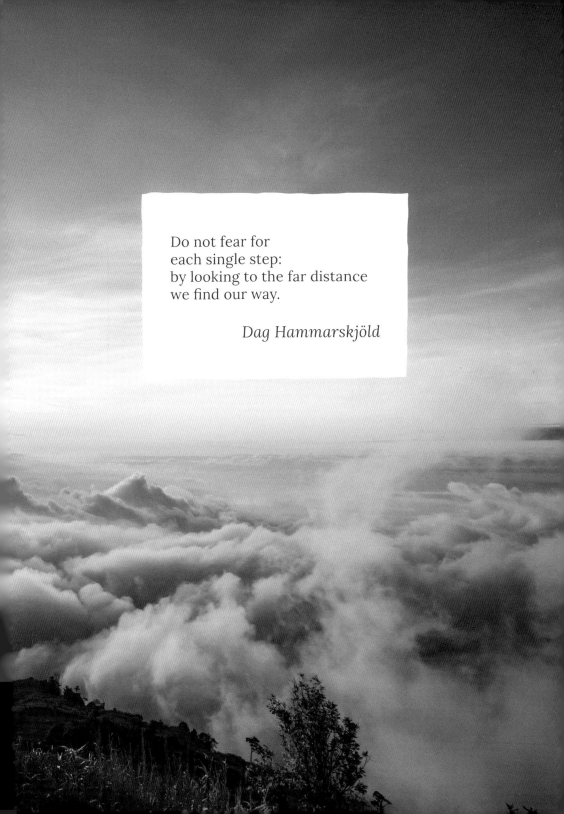

Do not fear for
each single step:
by looking to the far distance
we find our way.

Dag Hammarskjöld

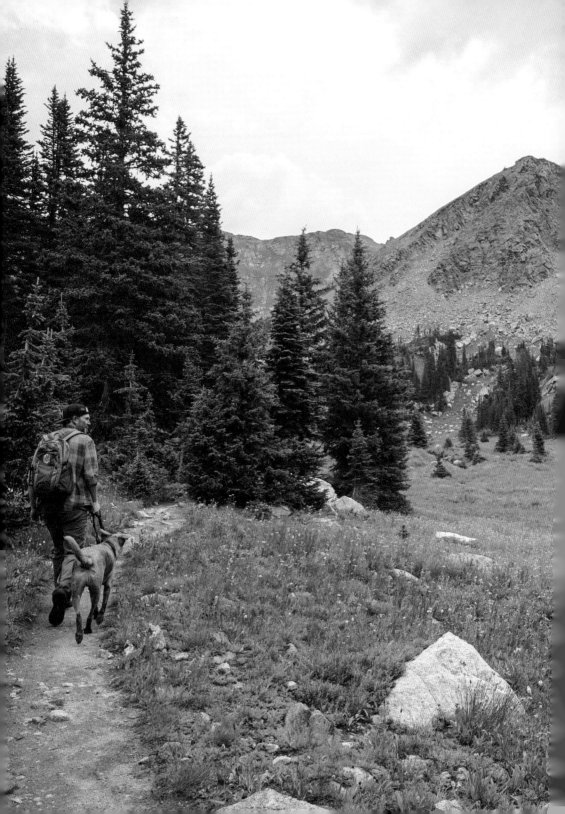

The Power of Inner Pictures

Many patients given a diagnosis of serious illness come to feel that their core task is transformation. Coming to terms with a diagnosis we often confront the question: what was, or is, wrong in my life? Deep down we feel that we cannot keep going in the same patterns. Something significant must change.

But change is not easy. The habits of a lifetime, the life history we carry in our bones, these things feel absolutely fixed. How do we create movement? How do we resolve on change and then act upon our resolution?

A picture of the future

Change is made possible by a picture of the future. In order to do things differently, we need a vision for ourselves: a picture of the future that we can live for. People who succeed in retaining or recovering hope despite a seemingly hopeless situation often tell of an inner picture that gave them strength.

If I keep doing things as I always have, will my experiences remain the same? Of course. So if I want my life to look and feel different, something will have to change. I will have to do things differently. This may be self-evident, but it is worth stating baldly, because change is so hard.

If I want to do things differently I need to be motivated by an inner picture of that difference: of who I am becoming, of how my life will grow.

93

Future visions bring strength

It is revealing to listen closely to the words of people who have survived disasters, imprisonment and extreme situations. Their testimonies have a common theme: they did not relinquish hope, because they held onto a vision of the future. Having purposes to live for, reasons to keep striving, a conviction that you will see people you love and do interesting things – these inner pictures of a fulfilling and inspiring future life give great strength.

Enlarging perspective

As well as becoming stuck in our habits, we can become narrow in our perspective over time. Broadening our perspective and considering unaccustomed outlooks with courage and trust is a step towards health. Living in openness towards what happens without preconceptions can help us to form new, sustaining thoughts. Perspectives may open up that are different from our previous ideas. A broader perspective can help us create fresh inner pictures: to literally see a new and different future.

Steiner on the power of inner pictures

Modern neurobiology or psychoneuroimmunology is confirming the effects of thoughts and feelings on bodily processes. But back in 1907, Rudolf Steiner gave a lecture on the power of inner pictures.

> The image works from the soul upon the organism, and the body's disposition for health is created by true pictures. False pictures also have an imprinting effect, engendering what we meet in psychological disturbances, which later become physical disorders. This is what really leads ultimately to pathological mental states. A person who

closes themselves off from the larger context of the world will not be able to fend off what they encounter. But by contrast it is impossible for someone who has informed themselves with great, true pictures to be deceived by false ones.[21]

Our collective picture of cancer

If our inner pictures have an effect on our physical reality, what impact is made by our culture's current picture of cancer? The media's portrayal of cancer has long emphasised death and tragedy rather than hope and recovery, despite the fact that more than half of all cancer patients do now recover.[22] As long as cancer is associated in the mind with death and dying, and as long as thoughts of recovery are suppressed in the media, we will collectively be creating negative inner pictures, along with their corresponding consequences.

Remember we can each create our own inner pictures. We do not need to absorb the prevailing view.

A story: Ingeborg's meditation

Ingeborg was a patient in our clinic. She had a major operation at the age of 85 to remove tumours that had amassed in her kidney. Ingeborg survived the operation but her body was struggling to recover from it. Her biochemical levels suggested she would die. But, astonishingly, she did not. And she continued to improve. The powers which support and configure life – 'life forces' if you like – got a grip again.

Later, she told us that for many years, during her daily walk through the woods, she always recited a meditation that she liked very much and had committed to memory.

She wrote the mediation down for us:

God in me,
my thanks to you
for the strength within
which here and now
brings me healing.

Transformation

If we ignore negative media portrayals and turn our eyes instead to life, we repeatedly see remarkable transformations. Life tells us that even when we receive a serious diagnosis, even when we are deep in ill health, it makes sense to prepare for both possibilities: living and dying.

Illness can lead us into a process of transformation, of making changes in our lives. We can start this process by cultivating pictures of the future. What will those pictures show for you?

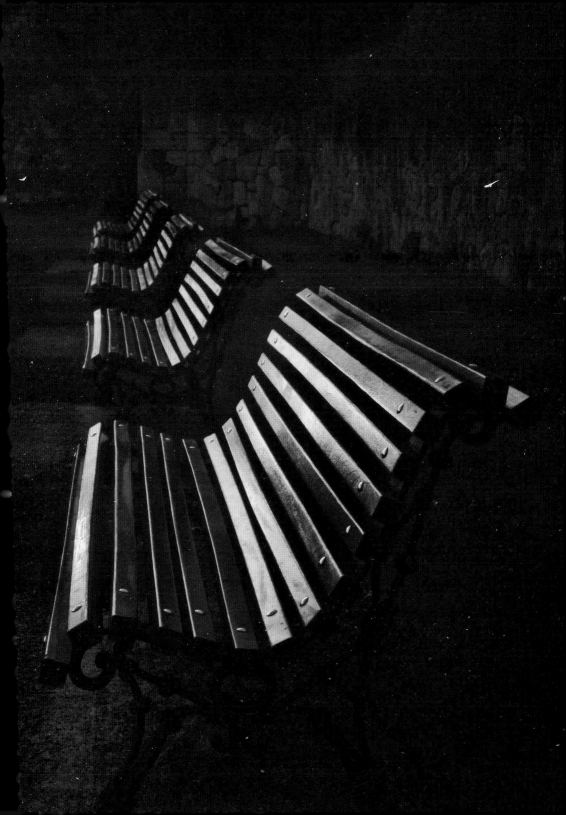

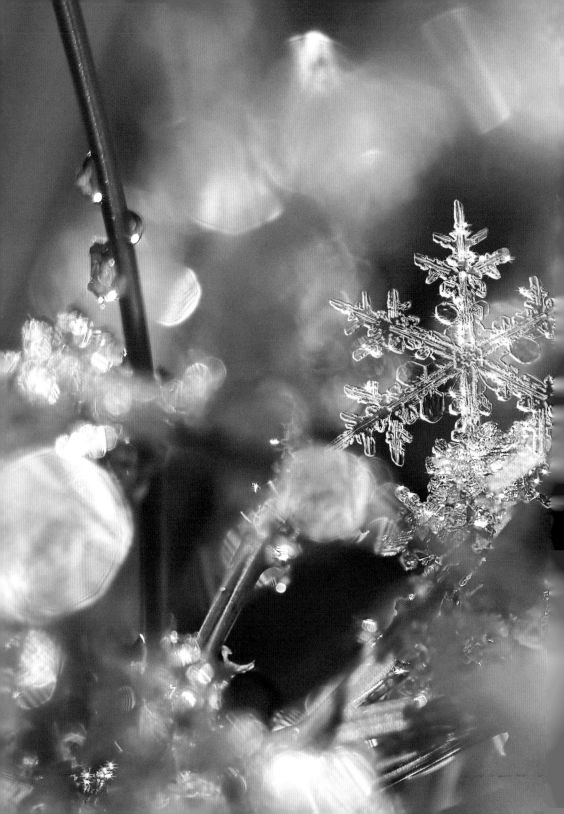

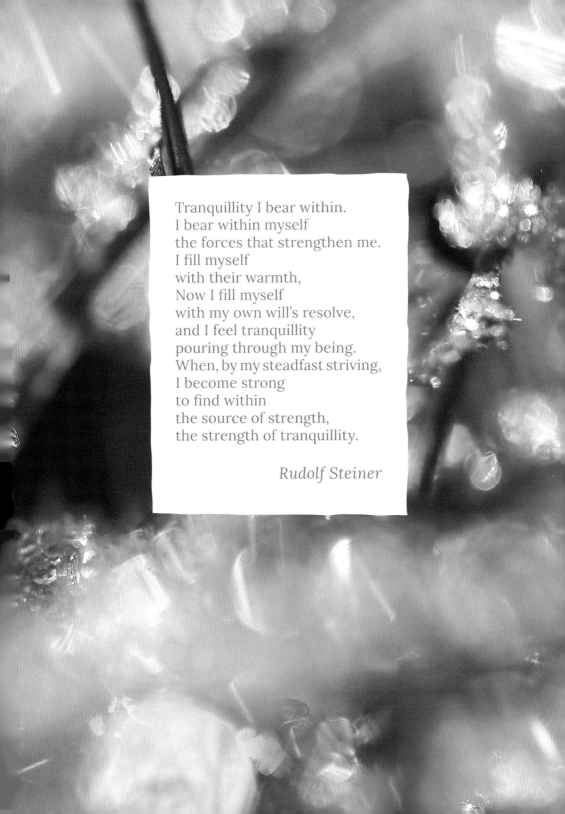

Tranquillity I bear within.
I bear within myself
the forces that strengthen me.
I fill myself
with their warmth,
Now I fill myself
with my own will's resolve,
and I feel tranquillity
pouring through my being.
When, by my steadfast striving,
I become strong
to find within
the source of strength,
the strength of tranquillity.

Rudolf Steiner

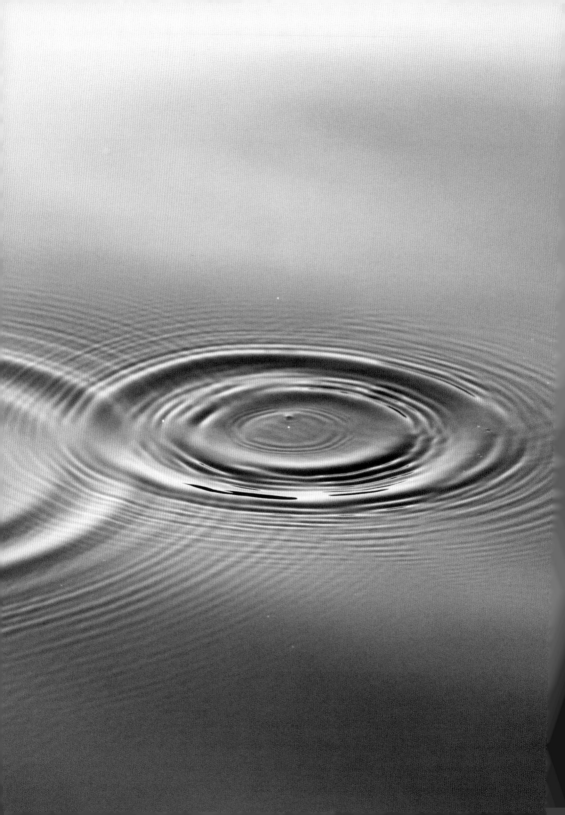

Tranquillity as Strength

Tranquillity as a path to health

Tranquillity can help stimulate the powers of healing and self-regeneration that always exist in us, even when we are struggling with illness.

If you are looking for ways to reshape your life, consider where and how you might cultivate tranquillity. It can be a path to health.

Questions: tranquillity

❋ What brings you peace and tranquillity?
❋ When did you last feel happily quiet inside?

Equilibrium between inner and outer worlds

Rudolf Steiner talked about the vital importance of tranquillity in human life, so we can reconnect with what is inside ourselves:

> In our life we find ourselves positioned between two forces: on the one hand the unfolding, ongoing sequence of events and realities,

which make the most varied impressions on us. Within us, at the same time, we have our own intrinsic strength. Even a superficial appraisal of life will show that we need to establish equilibrium between the events and facts that storm in upon us from all sides, and what unfolds within us. Having received a wealth of impressions in the business of daily life, we yearn for reflection, for solitude. We sense that a healthy life can only be found in the right equilibrium.[23]

Tranquillity is a precondition for coming back to ourselves, for recognising and perceiving ourselves again. Equally we need it in order to form the right decisions, and then to fully act on these decisions. Tranquillity or composure is a great help in all these sequential stages and processes.

Questions: why do we avoid peace?

When I give seminars on healing, and raise the importance of finding time and space for tranquillity, the responses are strong and almost unanimous:

* ❋ 'But I get no peace!'
* ❋ 'But there's always someone who needs me.'
* ❋ 'But there's too much to do: I sit down for a meal and immediately I see everything that still needs to be done, and then I leap up again and do it.'
* ❋ 'But when I try having some peaceful time, my head fills up with anxious thoughts. It's better to keep busy!'

Let's ask ourselves:

✳ What are we running from? What prevents us from meeting ourselves? What are we fearful of?

    Is it perhaps dying and death? Perhaps we know unconsciously that we will, ultimately, meet ourselves. In the end, the other demands, all that keeps us busy, will fall away and we will be faced with ourselves.

✳ With what stance would you wish to approach and meet yourself?

    If you can answer this question, please do so from a deep, heartfelt place, from the core of your being. If you already know the answer, you can start practising this stance today.

✳ How can you turn your stance for meeting yourself into daily habits and practices?

Is it selfish?

One reason many of us avoid taking time for tranquillity is we have internalised the idea that taking care of ourselves is selfish or egotistical.

✳ Is it selfish to withdraw from others for a while?

✳ Do you believe that taking time on your own for reflection is egotistical?

✳ When you plan your day and your week, juggling all the demands, are you regarding time with yourself as an indulgence, rather than a need?

Quiet and peace are essential for all human beings, especially when we want to make healthier changes in our lives.

A story: Sister Franziska's appointment with herself

Sister Franziska entered into her calling in part because she so highly valued time to reflect. But then, a woman of many talents, she found over time she had taken on numerous tasks and obligations in her order, and had almost no time for the quiet stillness that had brought her there in the first place. Increasingly she missed having time for herself. And it was difficult to push back against the tasks and obligations once she was established in the minds of others as the person responsible for them.

Then she found a solution: 'I say that I am sorry, I have no time at a certain point in the day because I already have an appointment. I don't tell anyone that this appointment is with myself!'

This is a solution that many of us need.

Make a regular appointment with yourself. Take time for quiet and peace.

In tranquillity and stillness we discover what is essential to us. It can seem contradictory when we are running from distraction to distraction that stillness is a source of energy, but we must trust that quietness is a different kind of activity, a deeper kind, and one we are liable to neglect – even to feel virtuous about neglecting. Tranquillity does not take time away; it replenishes us.

Times of calm peace and reflection also ensure that all your busy action at other times continues to follow your own unique path in life.

Let us be open to hearing what comes to us in tranquillity.

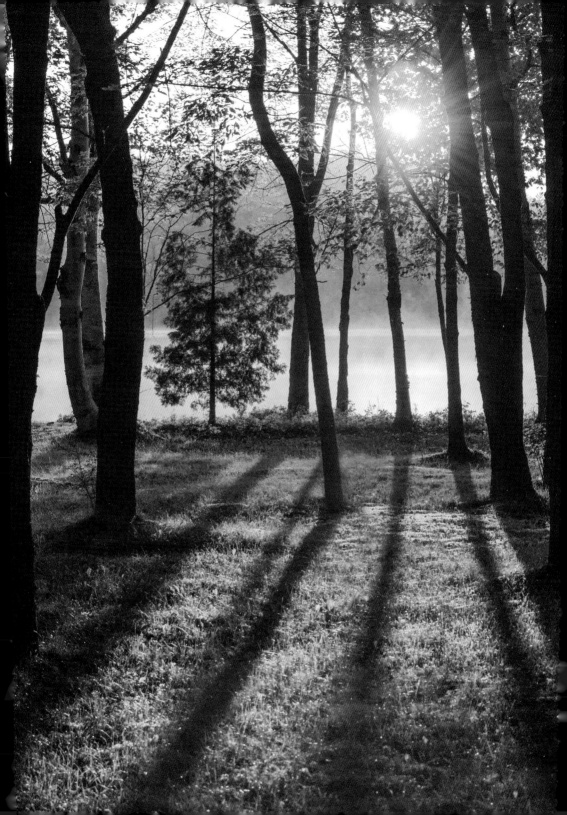

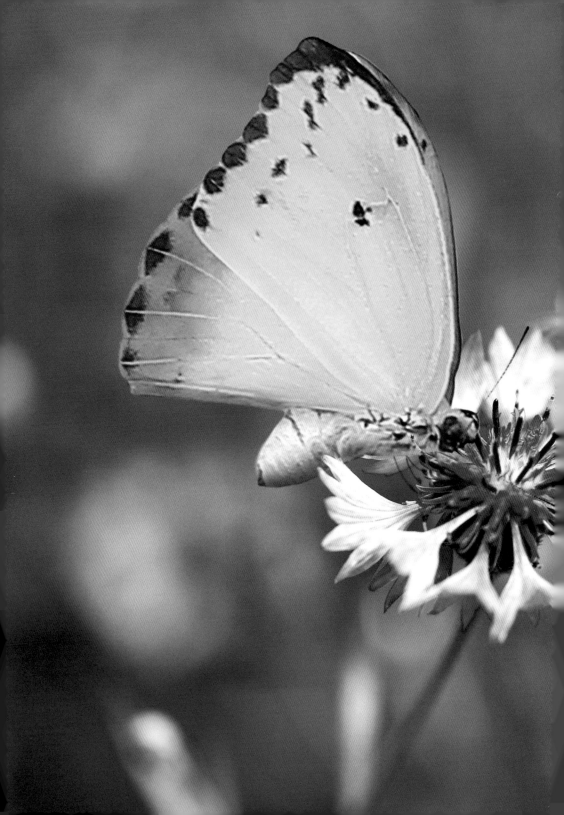

If caterpillars knew that they
would become butterflies,
they would live differently:
happily, confidently, hopefully.
Death is not the end.
The butterfly is the symbol of transformation,
metaphor for rebirth.
Life does not end but is altered.
The butterfly reminds us
that we are not entirely at home in this world.

Willi Hofsümmer

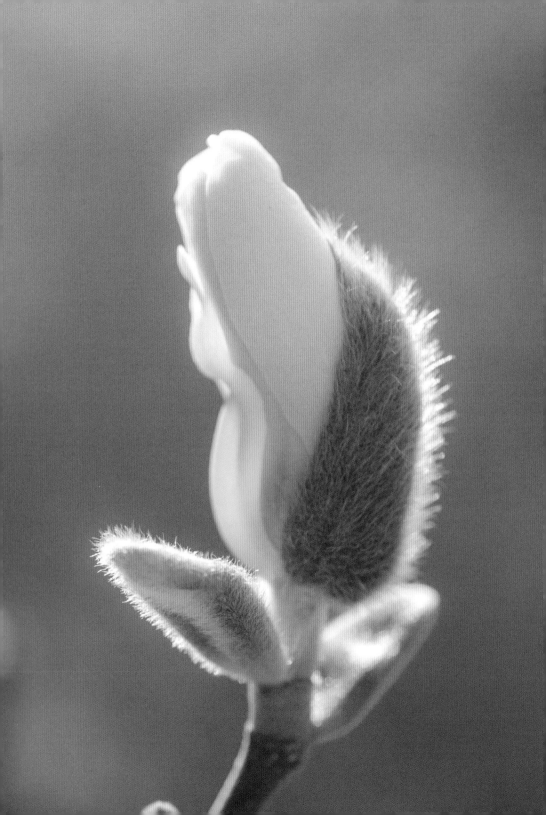

Death as Life's Assistant

Contemplating Death

We are all mortal: we face the fact that life will end. It is up to each of us whether to allow ourselves to think about this or push it away.

However paradoxical it may sound, an awareness that we are only a passing guest upon this earth can help us to focus on essentials, on what we wish to bring to the world from our own unique impulses.

Intensity

Sometimes I meet patients who have long made dying and death an integral part of their lives. It seems to me that these people live more intensely, precisely because they recognise that life might end any time.

In past ages, wise people thought that the art of living and the art of dying were one and the same. They taught that we live more fully if we acknowledge and accept death.

An old patient told me that she often finds herself thinking of the saying: 'Nothing is as certain as death, and nothing so uncertain as its date.'

Life requires death

Life is not possible without death. We see this in so many aspects of our being and the world around us. Think of cell biology, which looks at life at the level of its basic building blocks. Billions of cells die in our organism each day, and this is the only means for our body to renew itself. Our body needs the capacity to die in order to live.

If we wish to acquire and develop a new capacity, we have to leave old ideas and habits behind. Change is only possible if we do. Throughout our lives we come up against limits, boundaries, thresholds, transitions, places of transformation. It is a very common experience, at such transformative moments, to feel that we are completely incapable or that there are no options left open. We cannot imagine how this situation could ever shift. But then, so often, life shows us a positive way forward. Moving beyond an impasse requires that some of our assumptions or ways of seeing – which seemed essential – are discarded, and a new way of seeing arises that enables life to go forward. In this sense, too, we are only capable of life if we are capable of dying, capable of letting go.

Acknowledging fears of death

Whether consciously or not, thoughts about dying and death live in us. Do these thoughts bring us tranquillity or do they fill us with panic and alarm? If our response is panic and alarm, trying to work through these feelings is a good idea, as otherwise they will drain us of valuable life force and healing energy. But often we do not think we have any 'tools' to engage with thoughts of death, and instead we shut them out. Anxiety blocks our ability to integrate death and dying into our broad understanding of ourselves and our future. What we do not integrate costs us strength that is then no longer available for our life's work and our relationships, or for keeping us healthy.

There are two aspects of fear. When there is an immediate threat requiring quick action, fear can save our life by lending us adrenalin and strength and decisiveness. But fear, especially if it is ongoing and perhaps unwarranted, can also paralyse us and prevent us drawing on our creative presence of mind in the moment. It is important to square up to this kind of fear by acknowledging and investigating it. We need to put the thoughts and ideas making us fearful into words so we can check how valid they are in reality.

If you have a fear of death this may be because you are not yet prepared for dying. Our fears of death can also show us the ideas we carry about what death is and what comes after it. Thinking and talking about these fears can help us prepare for death and to develop our picture of death. Getting help and support from loved ones and professionals allows us to process our fears.

Can thinking about death be harmful?

I often meet people who have no wish to reflect on dying and death. They believe that these are negative thoughts, and will therefore do them no good. Unless you are ready to die, they say, you should focus on life.

This might be true at certain moments for one or another person. But most of us use this line of argument as a means of avoidance and I believe it can be harmful if it becomes a permanent defensive resolve. If we shut ourselves off from thinking of death, we deny ourselves vital opportunities for understanding and development.

I like the words of one of my seminar participants:

> The ability or willingness to reflect on death and dying has nothing to do with wanting to die. Nor does thinking about death make it more likely, as many fear. It's not about wanting to die, but about finding a sovereign composure towards everything life can bring or offer.

What is 'sovereign composure'? It means a calmness inside as we accept and acknowledge everything life presents to us.

Engaging with death and dying is usually a step into a deeper life. It can in fact give us energy for living.

A story: Bernhard's preparation for dying and for living

In the summer of 1985 my friend Bernhard, who was only 27 at the time, received devastating news. He had suffered a convulsion and as a result had a series of hospital tests. These revealed he had a glioblastoma, a brain tumour, and had no more than six months to live.

Bernhard accepted the seriousness of the diagnosis and made full preparations for the end of his life, seeking out texts to be read at his funeral, drafting an obituary and writing cards to be sent to his friends after he died.

At the same time, he maintained his connection with life. He had an open and independent mind, and was deeply imbued with a sense of wonder and respect for God in nature and the human being. This put his own pain and suffering in a larger context. In the forefront of his mind was a desire to help shape the world in positive ways. He was full of creativity.

Despite all expectations, he survived far beyond the six months given him: to the astonishment of medical professionals, he lived for another 27 years.

I was always amazed and grateful for Bernhard's openness to life's possibilities, and I feel his story confirms for me that an engagement with death and dying does not mean you want to die. Bernhard wrote his own obituary in the weeks after his diagnosis and he kept it on hand in his drawer for 27 years of fully involved life.

When family members won't talk about death

Many patients say that while they sense the importance of reflecting on death and dying, when they try to share thoughts with family members, they meet defensiveness and denial. Those around them don't like to allow the possibility of death, so they turn away from such discussions or shut them down. This can cause patients much psychological pain. They may feel very alone.

When death does come, family members who haven't talked about it may deeply regret that a chance for talking was missed, and realise that they themselves didn't take an opportunity to prepare for the loss that was coming. My experience has repeatedly been that when people are unable to engage with the issue of dying and death, an important developmental opportunity is lost. They miss out on conscious leave-taking and preparation for the other side of life.

If we do not broach the end of life in our conversations because we are clinging insistently to the idea of recovery, we will be poorly prepared, and the time we do have left with our loved one will be filled with anxiety. Last months and days need to be acknowledged as different and special. There needs to be a chance to express thanks for everything we have shared. Trying to carry on keeping everything the same as usual by not mentioning a possible end is a mistake.

I have listened with admiration to families and groups of friends succeed in discussing the imminent death of one member, sharing their thoughts, worries and questions. My perception has always been that discussion led to increasing peace and trust.

Trust

A patient who did not have long to live told me that she was intensely preoccupied with dying and death, and that while she thought about the end of her life, she kept inwardly hearing the words: 'Have trust.'

An exercise: the three mountain climbers and preparation

Imagine three mountain climbers getting ready for an alpine ascent in the Swiss Alps in October. They plan to stay in mountain cabins each night, but need to pack clothing.

The first climber, let's call her the optimist, packs only summer gear in her rucksack – t-shirts, shorts, sun hats – as it has been a warm September and she sees no reason to expect a change in the weather.

The second climber, who we will call the pessimist, believes that given it is October, the weather is bound to change for the worse, and he packs only winter gear: woollens, thermal leggings, a coat.

The third climber decides he cannot be sure what the weather will be, so he will try to cover all possibilities: one t-shirt, one woollen top, a sun hat and a warm hat.

* Now stop reading and try to imagine the feelings of each of these climbers as they set off. Who is comfortable? Who is relaxed?
* Then try to imagine the feelings of each after four days of walking in warm sunny weather. Who is comfortable? Who is relaxed?
* When a blast of wintery weather arrives, how would each of them feel?
* And finally, stop and consider: which of the three would you prefer to be?

This exercise shows what can be gained by preparing for all future possibilities. Once they have imagined the feelings of all three climbers, most people would prefer to be the one who accepts beforehand he can't know what the weather will be and so has thought about what he will need no matter what happens. The sense of being prepared for all possibilities brings equanimity. It means that the third climber can stop thinking about the weather and look about at the view. He is relaxed, physically comfortable, enjoying the present, able to adjust to what arises.

Each of us knows that death is one of our future certainties. If we have prepared for it, if we have thought through its implications, we can relax and enjoy the lives we have. Preparation for death can give us composure and strength for living.

Living with our mortality

Prior to the twentieth century, people considered it quite natural to prepare for dying and death, and to be ready for it throughout their lives. For example, they might have made their own shroud and have it ready in a drawer. People lived with a constant awareness of mortality. At the same time, many felt assured by their faith of eternal existence.

Some Buddhist monks turn their empty water glass upside down every night before they go to sleep. As they do it, they consider that they might die in the night. If they do indeed die in the night, the upturned glass shows they were ready for their journey.

When I was a child, my mother said evening prayers with us. She spoke of family members already in heaven, and the prayers asked us to live every day as if we might depart this life at any time.

These stories stand in contrast to modern culture, which also tends to be more atheistic. It is far more normal now to suppress thoughts of dying and death. But in moments of grief we can recognise a longing to bring our minds to the journey of the dead. We still need memorials, we need to think of those we've known who have passed away. Sometimes we still need to pray.

The three time zones

Dr Carl Simonton coined the idea of three time zones to help navigate the fears and anxieties of death and dying.

1. The first time zone runs from now to the time prior to dying.
2. The second time zone includes the last few hours of life and the process of dying itself.
3. The third time zone is the time after death.

We will all have different emotions about these different time zones, and you may find it helps to address each one separately.

❋ The first time zone usually makes people feel most anxious.
❋ Most of us ignore the second time zone; we want to deny it will arrive. It may be worrying us at some level but we put it out of mind.
❋ For some, the third time zone is still more horrendous to contemplate.

But these feelings are very individual.

We need to probe our ideas and pictures of each of these three zones, and then to work them through. For you, which zone feels most anxious? Which one feels most frightening? What are the possibilities for you in each of these zones?

Get help and support where you need it. It is possible to develop pictures of each of these zones that sustain our courage and trust.

Carl Simonton suggests to all of us, not just to those facing serious illness, that the most helpful inner stance is to have plans and desires for the next twenty years of life but at the same time to be ready to die today. We are not called upon to accept our illness and give up on living. We are not called upon to deny the possibility of death. We are best served by preparing for both life and death.

What Happens After Death?

Does a part of us continue after death? In the present-day western world, people find it difficult to imagine that there might be a part of themselves that is immaterial, immortal. The inscription on Albrecht Dürer's gravestone was: 'Here rests the mortal part of Albrecht Dürer.' This may now seem an odd expression to many. The idea that we are complex entities with both mortal and immortal elements has gone the way of Sunday hats and gloves. In a purely materialist understanding of the world, the whole of us ceases to exist when we die. Many people who feel that they and their loved ones have a soul or spirit nonetheless see the soul and spirit as dying with the body.

Questions: what do you believe?

* Do you believe each person has an immortal element?
* What do you think happens to consciousness as we die, and what happens to it after death?

But for a few of the patients I have talked to, death is a birth into a new and different world or existence. For these patients, joy can prevail over pain and grief even as they are dying.

Considering birth

If unborn babies had self-consciousness, and knew in advance what would happen to them at birth, they would surely regard birth as a death: the sacs surrounding them tear, the amniotic fluid in which they have so far lived flows away, the umbilical cord that has provided all nutrients is cut – everything they have experienced ends and they will never return to it. If they could conceptualise all this, birth would surely appear a frightening end to the life and self they've known.

But seeing birth as death would of course overlook the fact that new organs for life in a different environment have already developed: lungs for breathing air, eyes to perceive a world of colours and shapes, and much more. This potentially hopeless demise of birth is in truth the passage into life.

And perhaps there may be parallels in our perception of death, which likewise seems to rob us of our known existence. But perhaps it seems to rob us because we can only see it from an earthly or biological perspective. Perhaps we are making the same misunderstanding an unborn baby would make when considering birth.[24]

Is the process of birth one of dying? And that of dying one of birth? Novalis says:

> When a spirit dies it becomes a human. And when a human dies, they become a spirit.[25]

Near-death experiences

Reading about other people's near-death experiences can open up new ideas for us about dying, ideas that may have the effect of dissipating our fear and allowing us to consider the possibility of a transformed existence after death.

Cardiologist Pim van Lommel has researched the experiences of heart patients who have been resuscitated after their monitors showed them to be clinically dead. Around 18–20 per cent of resuscitated patients recall spiritual experiences, often reporting that their physical limitations dissolved. The distinction between space and time disappeared. Sometimes they report seeing the thoughts of other people or speaking to dead souls.

The great majority of people who have near-death experiences find that life alters radically for them after resuscitation. They report feeling less materialistic, less ambitious. They have little interest in personal power, prestige or fame. They are often much more selfless than before, more interested in relationships and in the spiritual aspects of life. Often, they have gained a certainty that their I, their soul, their consciousness, exists quite distinctly from their body's functions. When 'at death's door', they saw what was happening to them through different eyes and from a different perspective. Past, present and often even the future were perceived simultaneously.[26]

Stories: communication with the dead and dying

Gisela had a clear and beautiful dream about her long-dead father. He was carrying an armful of roses, and told her he was waiting for his wife and was so looking forward to seeing her.

The next day Gisela received the news that her mother had died unexpectedly.

She told me that this experience strengthened her trust in a world beyond the existence we can see and know.

* * *

Maria was accompanying sixteen-year-old Achim as he lay dying. She told me that each time she took her leave from him she would say, 'Hang on until I come again.'

One day, when Maria was shopping, Achim's grandfather was sitting with him in the hospital. Achim told him, 'I'm going home today.'

The grandfather replied gently that he wouldn't be discharged, but Achim seemed calm and certain.

Shortly after this, the grandfather could see Achim's physical condition was worsening. He said, 'Achim, I think we should call Maria and ask her to come now.'

Achim replied, 'I have called her already.'

Maria told me later that she had been standing with her supermarket trolley at the check-out when she clearly heard Achim calling her.

She rushed to the clinic, and was there, holding his hand, when he breathed his last.

* * *

Two sisters were sitting by their mother's death bed. They asked her to give them a sign when she reached the other side. Soon afterwards the mother passed away peacefully.

Some time later, one of the sisters had a clear and vivid dream in which she met her mother and spoke with her. Deeply moved, next day she went to see her sister to tell her about it. The other sister listened wide-eyed, then said that she had had exactly the same dream.

* * *

The Dalai Lama says we gain a different understanding of the world of spirit when we study stories of synchronicity like these ones.[27]

A sense of connection with people who have died

Rudolf Steiner spoke of cultivating a healthy relationship with the dead, and suggested it could resemble your connection with someone who has, say, emigrated to Australia. If we imagine there being no telephone or internet connection with Australia, and no means to get there, how would we nurture our relationship with the other person?

Most people reply, 'by thinking of them'.

Thinking with loving thoughts of those who have died maintains and honours a connection.[28]

Questions: surviving crises

Look back through your own life to times of crisis or trauma when your situation seemed bleak.

* How did you survive these times?
* What helped you?
* Where did those times of crisis lead?
* When and how did you know the crisis was over?

Often we can recognise that a situation that appeared hopeless later gave rise to some positive changes or development.

Reflecting on difficult times and our capacity to survive them can bring us trust and courage in the face of present uncertainty. We can recognise that help will come to us when we need it, that we are not alone nor forsaken.

As Dietrich Bonhoeffer put it, we are 'wonderfully protected by benevolent powers'.[29]

Heart knowledge

When considering the world of the spirit, trust in the wisdom of your heart, in what you feel to be true. Give yourself permission to believe and trust what your heart knows.

You cannot die alone

Elisabeth Kübler-Ross once talked in an interview about the strength of her conviction that we cannot die alone:

> You might send someone to the Moon in a space rocket, and they might go off in the wrong direction and travel around in space until they die in the rocket. But the people that person loved who died before them will always be expecting them. Those people will always be there. You can't die alone.

When the interviewer objected that she couldn't know this for sure, she went on:

> For me this isn't a matter of faith but a fact of knowledge. Anyone who is unafraid and really wants to study these things, can verify them. The beautiful thing is that it is true for everyone on earth. If you collected cases of two- and three-year-old children who can tell you what they experience at the moment of death, even you would grasp that this is true: two and three year olds, after all, haven't read any books, and aren't trying to prove anything. They don't lie about these things.

When the interviewer asked her if she was afraid of dying, she replied:

No, not at all! I'm looking forward to it! ... Life is far, far harder than dying.[30]

Illness calls us back to our life's purpose

The artist André Heller once said that every person comes to Earth as a 'blueprint' rather than in finished form. 'I, André Heller,' he said, 'have decided to be the best realisation of the André Heller blueprint that is possible for me!'[31]

Surely we all harbour a secret desire to be the best possible realisation of the blueprint of ourselves. But we may well have lost sight of this blueprint, perhaps feeling that perfecting it, or even being true to it, is beyond our reach.

Illness can reconnect patients with lost visions and ideals, helping us get back in touch with the inherent qualities that should resound through us. We can suddenly recognise that we have become something we didn't intend – not our true selves – and can begin to think about how we might return to what we hold sacred, or to what is intrinsic to us.

Surely the deeper meaning of health could be connected with becoming who we really are. And illness could be seen, partly at least, as losing sight of our intrinsic being, perhaps because we have been trying to be what others wanted, or because we lost touch with our true heart and mind, or because we haven't yet been able to find our real calling or destiny.

Perhaps illness is not something pitted against us, but can help us follow our life's deeper purpose. Dr Carl Simonton says:

Illness is a messenger of love, seeking to help me become more truly myself.

Questions: what gifts has illness brought you?

Illness is understood as an affliction, as something we would always wish to escape. Yet it is also true that many people who have come through long spells of illness recognise that they also have positive feelings about what happened to them. Illness brought with it insight, or time, or a different point of view that they would not now want to be without.

Recognising that there will also be many negative aspects, what are the positive aspects of illness in your own life?

* Has illness meant you have more time for yourself? More time with your own thoughts?
* Do you value your time more?
* Have some things in your life become more important than before?
* Have your priorities changed?
* Are there new people in your life now, for whom you feel grateful?
* Have some relationships grown more intense and alive while others have faded into the background?
* Do you now take more care before saying yes, and do you allow yourself to say no more often?
* Do you feel you have learned new things? Gained new perspectives?
* A final and most important question: Are you more in touch with yourself now, or through illness have you grown further away from what you feel to be your true nature?

Returning to our own deeper purpose

In his poem 'I Am Not I', Juan Ramón Jiménez insists we are more than what we see and measure:

> I am the one ...
> who keeps tranquil silence when I speak,
> who meekly forgives when I hate, ...
> who will stand upright when I die.[32]

Preoccupation with the theme of death and dying not only releases powers in us that support the body in maintaining health and recovery, but also helps us to reflect on what is really important in life. Awareness of our finite lives allows us to attend to the realisation, here and now, of our life's plan.

Accepting uncertainty

Uncertainty about whether there is a life after death is a healthy response. We do best when we accept uncertainty and don't resort to replacing it with fixed, materialist certainties that shut down possibility.

From loss to gain

Death is often associated with pictures of loss and ending, but can we, inside ourselves, replace these pictures with images of a new beginning, of transformation? People who have had near-death experiences have experienced their I, soul, and consciousness to be in an excellent state despite their body having no signs of life. Perhaps illness, that failure of our physical being, is our chance to see what there is inside us that goes beyond the confines of the physical world.[33]

No one wants to die. Even people who want to go to heaven don't want to die to get there. And yet death is the destination we all share. No one has ever escaped it. And that is as it should be, because Death is very likely the single best invention of Life. It is Life's change agent. It clears out the old to make way for the new. ... Remembering that I'll be dead soon is the most important tool I've ever encountered to help me make the big choices in life. Because almost everything – all external expectations, all pride, all fear of embarrassment or failure – these things just fall away in the face of Death, leaving only what is truly important. Remembering that you are going to die is the best way I know to avoid the trap of thinking you have something to lose. You are already naked. There is no reason not to follow your heart.[34]

US entrepreneur Steve Jobs

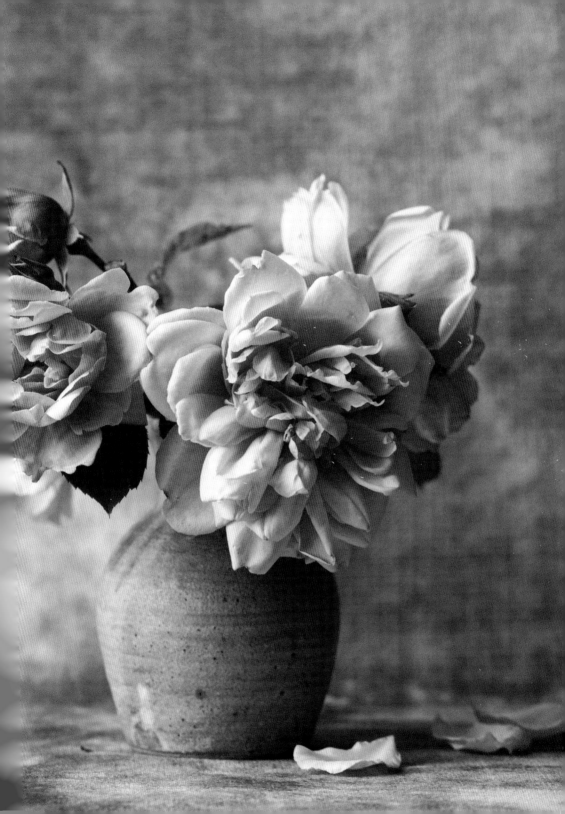

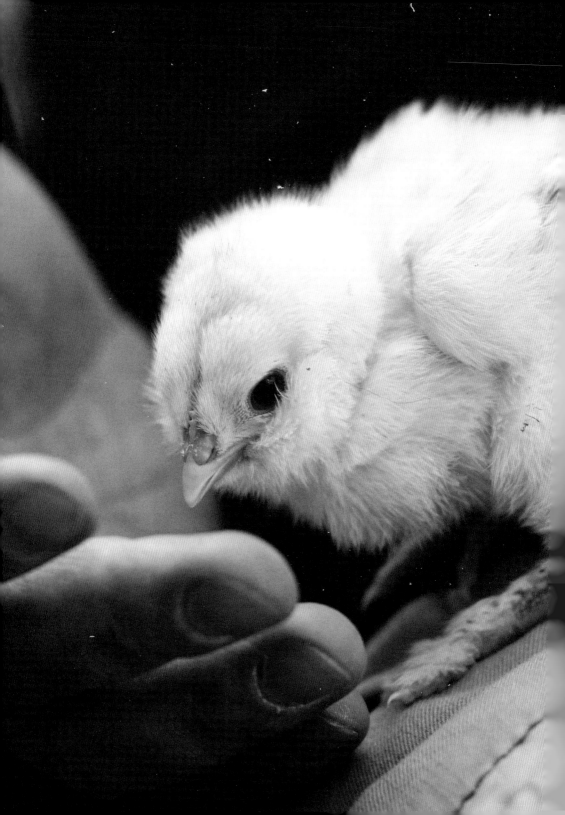

As I began to love myself I found that anguish and emotional suffering were only warning signs that I was living against my own truth. Today I know this is AUTHENTICITY.

As I began to love myself I stopped craving for a different life, and I could see that all that surrounded me was inviting me to grow. Today I call it MATURITY.

As I began to love myself I quit stealing my own time, and I stopped designing huge projects for the future. Today I only do what brings me joy and happiness, things I love to do and that make my heart cheer, and I do them in my own way and in my own rhythm. Today I call it SIMPLICITY.

As I began to love myself I refused to go on living in the past and worrying about the future. Now, I only live for the moment, where everything is happening. Today I live each day, day by day, and I call it FULFILLMENT.

We no longer need to fear arguments, confrontations or any kind of problems with ourselves or others. Even stars collide, and out of their crashing, new worlds are born. Today I know THAT IS LIFE!

*Charlie Chaplin**

* These words are also attributed to Kim McMillen.

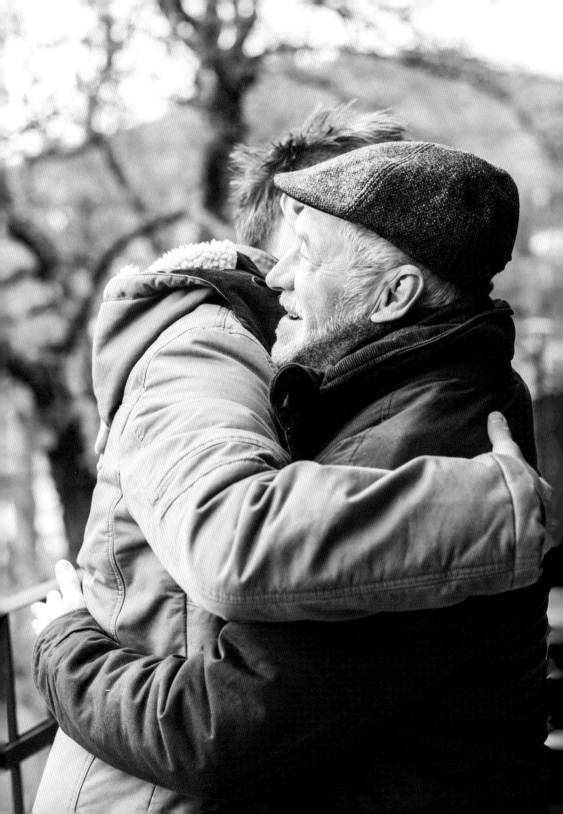

The Healing Power of Love

Everybody needs love and connection

Caryle Hirshberg has done research on cancer in animals and reports that malignancies grow more slowly in animals receiving more care, attention and play.

We know very well from epidemiological statistics that loneliness among humans creates significant health problems and leads to poorer treatment outcomes.

What is at work here? Something in our social relations affects us in real ways, though we cannot see it or medically account for it. This factor is not based on any material substance. Most research into health and treatments, whether for humans or other animals, does not consider it.

In the thirteenth century, Frederick II, Holy Roman Emperor, tried to investigate the 'primordial language' – he wanted to discover which language children would speak if they weren't taught any other. He separated babies from all human life, except that they were given the bare essentials of feeding and changing. They weren't allowed to hear a single word of human language. Rather grimly, he discovered that 'children could not live without clappings of the hands, and gestures, and gladness of countenance, and blandishments.'

Humans are fundamentally social beings – we need connection with

131

other people to live. We need it every bit as much as we need food. Language, the Word, is life and spirit. And without love we are nothing.

The heart

> Heaven is neither above or below, neither to the right nor to the left, heaven is to be found exactly in the centre of the bosom of the man who has faith.[35]
>
> – Salvador Dali

If asked which bodily organ love is rooted in, we are unlikely to say the spleen, liver, lungs or kidneys. Traditionally it is the heart.

What qualities or attributes do we assign to the heart?

* Strength
* Generosity
* Warmth
* Joyfulness
* Gratitude
* Enthusiasm
* Sympathy

Cancer can appear in many places in the body – except for one that is almost never affected by it. I have never yet met a cancer patient who had a tumour of the heart.

Is this because the heart embodies qualities that are oppositional to those of the tumour process? Is it possible that the qualities we associate with a loving heart (a courageous heart, a trusting heart, a cheerful heart...) might be a wonderful source of sustenance for our immune system? What quality is it that flows through the heart and configures its biochemistry in such a way that tumours do not form there?

Questions: joy and enthusiasm

❋ What in your life thus far has made your heart leap with joy or enthusiasm?

❋ How could you enliven the experience and feeling of joy and enthusiasm within you now? As you move forward?

❋ Can you nurture these feelings in your life, as you would nurture a germinating plant?

Heart science

It is interesting to learn what modern science has discovered about the heart. The brain is vital of course, but it takes its lead from the heart, which creates the strongest electric field in our body – a hundred times more powerful than the brain. Likewise, the heart creates our body's strongest magnetic field, five-thousand times stronger than that of the brain. We live in a world of electrical and magnetic fields. Modern research shows that through these fields the human heart is energetically connected with all physical reality.[36]

These findings accord to an astonishing degree with the traditional wisdom of ancient cultures. According to the Norwegian Ole Martin Hoystad, in Arabic and Islamic culture the heart is thought to be the 'organ of God':

> To heed the will of God, you are meant to follow the dictates of your heart, since that is where God manifests, speaking to us through it. The Sufis have their own teachings about the heart, as a channel of communication between man and God. One should enquire into one's heart: to know God one must know one's own heart.[37]

The HeartMath Institute in California has carried out research on the intelligence of the heart. This has shown that the heart has its own intelligence, which is in some ways superior to that of the brain.

Also, the cells of the heart are particularly long-lived. They have a double nuclei, and do not die and renew at the rate of other cells in our bodies.

When love or esteem streams towards someone, an invisible but nevertheless perceptible force field is created which also radiates to the person's wider surroundings. Mystics of all traditions have described this phenomenon, including the Sufi Master Hasrat Inayat Khan, who writes:

> A heart's honest feelings can penetrate another's heart; they speak silently by expanding on all sides, so that the atmosphere a person spreads around them announces their thoughts and feelings.[38]

If we wish to heal our body, or if we resolve to create peace in our families, communities and between nations, we must connect with the field that connects everything, and this is precisely the realm of the heart.

Our heart is a great, warm, powerful healing resource inside each one of us, and its strength grows rather than shrinks with use.

A story: describing your own work

A patient who came regularly to my art therapy studio looked at the painting she had just done and said, with some detachment, 'That isn't at all bad!'

Then she laughed at her own words and went on: 'It would be much better to say what it is, not what it isn't. Why don't I just say, "That's good!"?'

Questions: do you love yourself?

* Can you engage lovingly with yourself?
* Can you accept yourself with all your failings and flaws?
* Can you recognise that each of us is on a path of development?
* Can you love yourself simply as you are?

Self-love as Aquinas described it

Thomas Aquinas described love for oneself as the *forma et radix* – the vessel and root – of all love. Saint Augustine proposed a fourfold love: the love for God, the love for oneself, the love for another and the love for one's body.

Much later in ecclesiastical history, Calvin and Luther gave the idea of 'self-love' a different, more egotistic, disparaging meaning. When I speak of loving oneself as a source of creative and healing energy, I am speaking of it as Aquinas intended.

Questions: loving oneself

Many of us have understanding for others, yet treat ourselves unlovingly. Most people endorse the Christian principle of 'Love thy neighbour as thyself', but the 'loving thyself' bit tends to gets lost.

* How do I practise love for myself?
* What would this involve?

* I may bow before the God in you, but can I respect the God in myself?
* Am I aware that the divine lives in me?
* What would it mean in practice to relate respectfully both to others and to oneself?

Love, as all parents know, can also involve consistency and firmness, in order to address bad habits.

A story: Anita Moorjani's recovery through self-love

Anita Moorjani, author of *Dying to be Me*, was in a coma, dying from lymphoma and had a near-death experience. She recovered rapidly, and believes her recovery was due to the insights she gained from her near-death experience. She believes her illness was caused by fear, lack of authenticity and lack of self-love.

> I wanted to please everyone and was anxious about people's poor opinions, whoever they might be. I tired myself out trying to prevent people thinking badly of me, and over the years I lost myself because of it. I became completely detached from the person I was or who I wished to be, because everything I did was geared to gaining approval and praise from all.

After her near-death experience she felt a moment of letting go: 'When I was ready to let go, I received what was really mine. I recognised that this is always the greatest gift.'[39] It was also important for her 'to gain an awareness that I am far more than my biology, that I am infinitely greater than that.'[40]

When asked about her recovery she speaks of:

> ...one of the best-kept secrets of our time. Love for oneself is enormously important. ... I cannot remember ever having been encouraged to value or esteem myself. The idea would never even have occurred to me, and is generally regarded as egotism. But my near-death experience showed me that this was the key to my recovery.

> [This also means] being aware how important it is to nourish my own soul, to accept my needs and not always put myself last. This enables me to stay true to myself at every moment, and to treat myself with absolute respect, friendliness and kindness. In this way also I can look without judgement at what can be seen as my flaws, imperfections and mistakes, seeing these as an opportunity to perceive and experience things with unconditional love, and to learn.[41]

Moorjani contrasts self-love with selfishness.

> Selfishness arises from lack of self-love. ... During my near-death experience I had a sense that judgement, hatred, jealousy and fear come from those who do not recognise their true stature. ... If we were encouraged to express our true being, it seems to me that we would all be very loving beings, and would be better able to express our unique qualities and give them to the world. ... If we stopped judging ourselves, we would immediately have less need to judge others. We would begin to perceive their real perfection. The universe is contained within us and what we experience outwardly is only a reflection of that inner world.[42]

Making choices about our time

Sometimes we have made choices that lead us away from what we really want and need. We bite off more than we can chew, get immersed in battles we think we have to fight to the end and win, we get lost in the details, and we lose sight of ourselves and our priorities. Sometimes we need to let go and return to what matters most.

We live in an economy driven by hurry, stress and seeming lack of time. This may lead to us 'just functioning': − not thinking, but responding in knee-jerk fashion to outer demands. And in doing so we can lose sight of ourselves and our own self-care.

Big rocks first

A teacher of time management showed his audience an empty bucket. He poured in sand and gravel, then held up a container holding rocks the size of tennis balls. 'Can I fit these in?' he asked. It was immediately clear he could not. The bucket was nearly full already.

He tipped out the sand and gravel and started again. First he put the rocks into the bucket. It already looked almost full.

He held up the sand and gravel. 'Can I fit these in?' he asked. The audience were unsure. He poured the sand and gravel in, where it settled among the bigger stones.

'What was I trying to demonstrate?' he asked.

Someone called out, 'The bucket is like our schedule. We think it's full but you can always squeeze more in!'

'No, that's not it,' replied the professor. 'The bucket *does* get full. What I wanted to show was that if you don't put the big stones in first, you won't find space for them. The big stones are the things in life that are especially important: your family, your health, what inspires and fulfils you. If you don't put the big stones in first, your time gets filled with the little stuff, and there's no room left for what really matters.'

Questions: self-love and self-care

It's important to take time to find out what is really important to you.

* What connects you lovingly to life?
* Can you surround yourself with these things?
* What is getting in the way of these things?

Thinking about the following questions can help us nurture the healing forces within ourselves:

* How do you show yourself love and respect?
* What does this mean in terms of daily or weekly activities and practices?
* Can you make space and time in your life for the things that are most important to you?
* Is there anything you do each day that is not required of you by others, and is not enforced by you, but that you do in inner freedom? Something you deeply want to do?

Here is a list created by one of my seminar groups. These are the ways they wanted to show care for themselves in future. This list might help you as you think through the questions above.

❋ Take more time for myself
❋ Learn to value, love and spoil myself
❋ Give myself gifts
❋ Find a strong balance between relaxation and work
❋ Fulfill my emotional needs as far as possible
❋ Attend to myself with respect, that is, listen to my inner voice
❋ Learn to say 'No': acknowledge my boundaries and limits
❋ Stand up for myself: say 'Yes' to myself
❋ Accept help
❋ Forgive myself and others
❋ Feel happy in the moment
❋ Feel gratitude for things (still) being as they are
❋ Decide not to seek harmony if it requires self-suppression
❋ Accept my illness without resignation

Any one of these acts is a significant step. Is there an idea here you would like to bring into your own daily life?

Self-love and self-knowledge

Love for oneself makes it possible to perceive, accept and know ourselves. And this in turn is the precondition for determining who we wish to be. When we determine this we can figure out how to change from the core of our being, authentically.

Without self-love, it is very difficult to perceive and know ourselves. And it will always be too arduous to enact the knowledge and resolve to be who we wish to be. Loving ourselves allows our full, healthy being to develop.

A story: where to find wisdom

There is an Indian legend that speaks of wisdom pervading the world.

A long time ago the gods realised it would be dangerous if people discovered the wisdom of the universe before they were ready for it. They decided to conceal it in a place where it would not be found until human beings had matured enough to understand it.

One of the gods proposed hiding it on the highest mountain. But the others calculated that human beings would climb every mountain before long, and this would not be a safe enough hiding place. Another god proposed putting the wisdom of the universe in the deepest ocean. But still the gods were worried that people might come across it too soon.

At last the wisest of the gods made this suggestion: 'I know what is to be done. Let us hide the wisdom of the universe inside human beings themselves. They will only look for it there when they are ready for it, for to find it they must take the inward path.'

The other gods were pleased with this suggestion and so they concealed the wisdom of the universe inside human beings, where it cannot be found until we are ready.

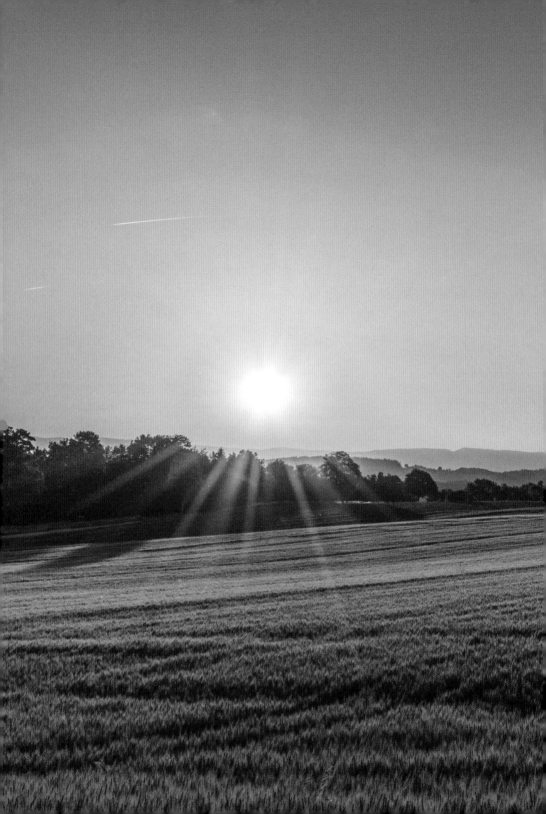

Mine are not the years time took from me,
mine are not the years that may still come,
mine is the moment, and when I tend to it,
then he who made eternity is mine.

Andreas Gryphus

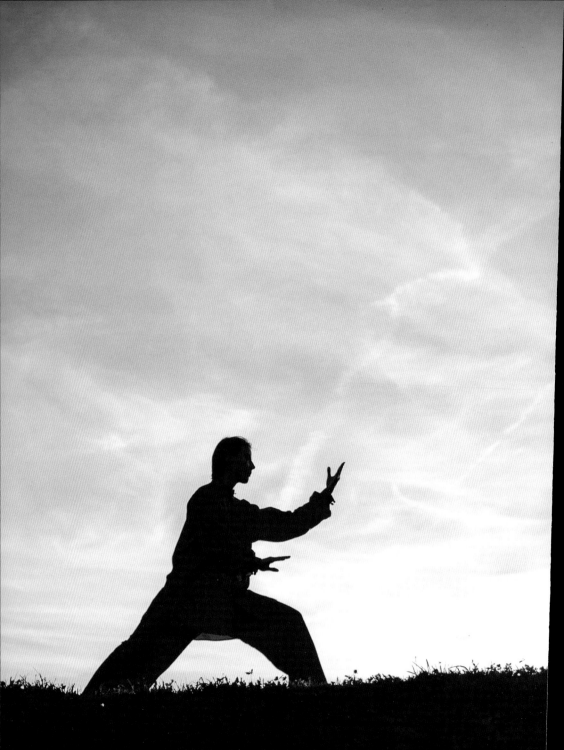

Looking for Light in the Darkness

Illness as a fight

When diagnosed with serious illness, we hear a lot about battles and fighting. This is so often the metaphor people unthinkingly call upon with all illness, but especially when talking about cancer: 'He lost the battle with cancer.' 'Help her fight cancer.'

Let's think about battles and fighting. Is this imagery helpful for you?

An exercise: what does fighting mean to you?

Form a sentence about yourself that starts with the words:
  'I fight…'

Consider how it feels for you to use those words. People have very different responses to the idea of fighting. What are your responses?

Write down your sentence (or imagine writing it).

What word follows 'fight'?

Two of the most common words to follow 'I fight...' are 'for' and 'against'. You may have used one of these words yourself. Even if you haven't used the words, do you have a sense of whether your words describe you fighting for or against something?

Or perhaps your answer indicates that you will not fight at all.

Where to use our energy

For some people affected by grave illness, fighting or battling is an existential need, an inner imperative. Others are overwhelmed by the idea of fighting on top of surviving. We are all different individuals, and a particular strategy can be helpful for one person but not for another. Among those who do use an image of fighting, there will be some for whom the noise of battle may drown out everything else, who lose sight of themselves. Battling can lead to a narrowing of focus, a fixation on the end result. For this reason some feel the imagery isn't helpful for them, and prefer to say 'I am nurturing my health.' Many patients find that the idea of 'fighting' comes with a great deal of pressure, which they would prefer to do without.

Battling is associated with huge exertion and requires a great deal of energy. For you, 'fighting' may be the best way to use it, but do stop and consider. There are many ways to use this energy.

If you are 'fighting', are you striving *for* or *against*? You might object that it's all words, that fighting for health is fighting against illness. But is it really the same? I think the distinction is important. The words 'for' and 'against' create different qualities in the mind. Political upheavals that only battle against an authority, with no thought and energy devoted to what they are battling *for*, lead to chaos. When our vision is focused entirely on being 'against', it bears no power to shape the future.

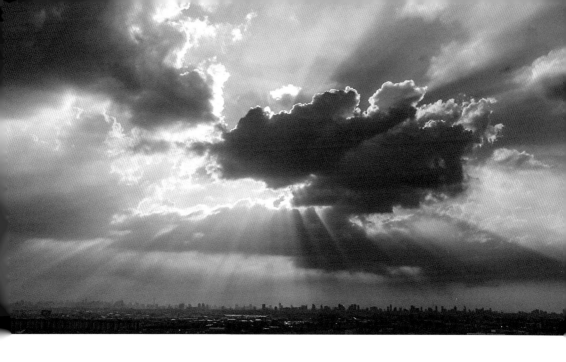

Focus on light not darkness

That which we think about magnifies in our lives. When we are ill, our thoughts can become crowded by shadows. We need mental imagery that helps us turn towards health and light. Our thoughts have more power than we perhaps expect.

If you are able to turn your thoughts from fighting *against* the illness to fighting *for* health, you may feel a more positive energy from this change of focus.

The shock of diagnosis with a serious illness can be compounded by a sense of gloom, as if one is plunged into a dark cloud that becomes the whole world, and one is filled with despair and hopelessness. Imagine a mountain climber who is lost in a heavy, dark cloud, and cannot see which way to go. We all know that endless views and sunshine lie beyond the clouds. And the light is always present in illness too.

Illness and health dwell side-by-side inside us, as do light and shadow, trust and doubt. The darker the shadow, the brighter the light.

No darkness exists without light. Perhaps what we now see as the darkness in our lives, we will come to understand as shadows cast by a light we could not recognise.

A story: the old woman and the cracked pot

Once upon a time there was an old woman who fetched water in two big pots hanging from the ends of a pole that she carried across her back. One pot had a crack, and the other was flawless. The perfect pot could always carry a full load of water, but the cracked pot leaked. By the time the old woman walked home from the river, the cracked pot was always half empty. The perfect pot was very pleased with itself; the cracked pot was ashamed of its flaw.

After two years of this failure every day, the cracked pot said to the old woman, 'I am so ashamed of my crack. Water is lost through it all the time you are trudging home!'

The old woman smiled and replied, 'Haven't you seen the flowers blooming all the way along the path from the river? They grow on one side, but not the other. I knew of your leak, so I sowed seeds, and now you water them every day as we step along.'

Decide what to focus on

We have the freedom to decide what we will focus on, what we will give our precious attention to. Not only the freedom, but also the capacity to perceive what lives in our mind and spirit, and how this affects us. We might compare our mind with a radio: it broadcasts the wavelength that we ourselves choose.

I myself decide what programmes I watch or listen to, which items of news I read, the books I want to immerse in. I myself decide how to fill my mind.

What we focus our attention on will grow within us.

The strength to fight out of our own darkness may feel lacking. But help comes from many quarters. We don't have to do everything alone. It is up to each of us whether we ask for help, and whether we accept it when it is offered.

A story: letting go of dark thoughts

A participant in my seminar told us about her experience of receiving a bad test result. All kinds of dark thoughts started crowding in on her. The nurse who was with her saw this and said, very directly: 'Let the spirit in again!'

The woman described taking a deep breath, and feeling that she could let the dark thoughts go.

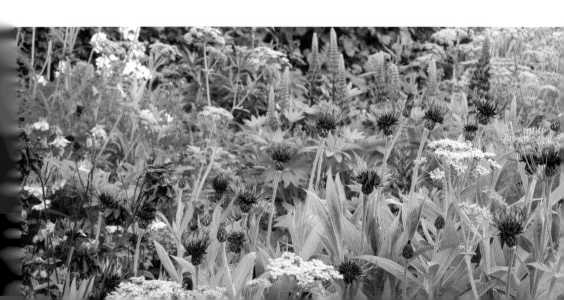

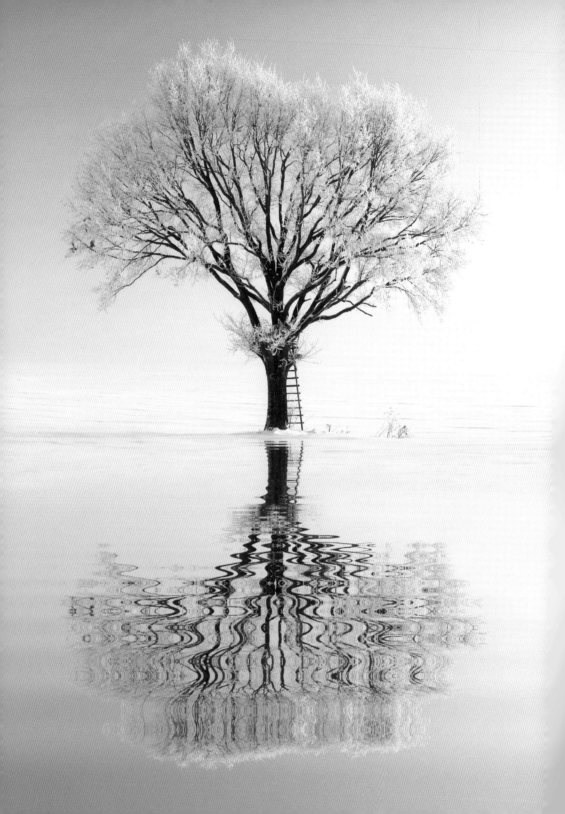

The Angel of No

A potent angel comes, and lo
courageously he utters 'No'!

A warrior angel standing tall
upon his own two feet. His call
is clarion bright like brilliant day,
delighting in the honest words we say.

A potent angel comes, and lo
courageously he utters 'No'!

This 'No!' means yes to risk, and not
just doing what seems advisable
to others. Far harder than an easy nod
and bending to the common will.

A potent angel comes, and lo
courageously he utters 'No'!

Jutta Richter

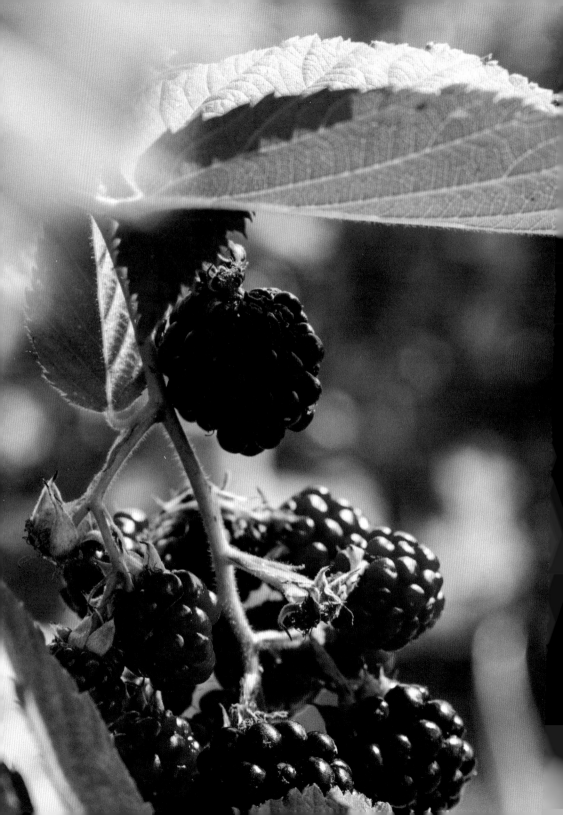

The Healing Potential of Autonomy and Authenticity

Caught in situations we don't want

It often happens that, perhaps out of a false idea of love, we get involved in a scenario or even a whole life that we never really wanted to be part of. Why do I end up doing things I don't want to do? How can I change my circumstances?

Most of us are familiar with this conundrum. Most of us have, at times, found ourselves in positions we've ended up in rather than chosen, and which do not feel right for us. The feeling of these situations is that we are standing a little outside ourselves.

In such situations, life is asking us to unpack a very specific little word. It is the word we need if we lovingly attend to ourselves and our own boundaries – which we must do to nurture our health.

The word is: 'no'.

An exercise: thinking 'no' but saying 'yes'

Recall a situation when life faced you with a question, and you felt the answer immediately, with great clarity and without doubt: 'No!' And yet your mouth opened and you heard yourself saying 'Yes.' Can you picture any particular instances when this has happened? Perhaps think about situations you are in right now that you would rather not be in, or commitments you have coming up that you wish you didn't have to follow through.

Take time to examine situations like this that you can bring to mind.

* In the initial moment when the situation was developing, what motivated you to change your instinctive answer?
* What were your different feelings at the time?
* Who else was involved?
* What thoughts twisted your crystal-clear 'no' into a 'yes'?

Pursuing this trail can be a helpful way to meet your own views of the world, your more or less unconscious ideas and assumptions. Try to put these thoughts and assumptions into words. Perhaps they will start something like this:

* Good neighbours always...
* It's my job to be the one who...
* I don't like to disappoint...
* It's best if we avoid...
* I don't want to fall out with...
* If I don't meet expectations then...

Once you have put words onto your motivations, ask yourself whether the ideas and assumptions that caused you to turn the 'no' into a 'yes' are life-enhancing?

I suspect that in the great majority of cases, you will be

uncovering habits of thought, of feeling and of dealing with others that are not healthy. They may be making life easy in the short-term but they have negative long-term effects.

Perhaps, for example, we say 'yes' for the sake of short-term peace. If we do things for the sake of 'peace', there will actually be no peace inside us: there can be no peace when we overlook our own inner voice.

Agreeing to, say, a social event when you know you really need time to yourself might forestall an argument, but it means going without the rest and reflection your inner voice is asking for.

Challenging our assumptions

When we find the courage and assurance to stand up for what we feel beyond doubt to be the right course of action, both we ourselves and those around us can develop in a healthy way. When I state my boundaries and needs clearly, others will be free to state their own, and to make different plans from me where they need to.

Some of us believe, deep inside, that if we don't meet others' expectations, we will no longer be loved. But love that is heavily conditional, conditional indeed on you not meeting your own needs, is damaging.

It is worth scrutinising the ideas and assumptions that lead us away from our own selves.

- ❋ Are these ideas absolute?
- ❋ Does everyone else live by them?
- ❋ Are they true in all cases?
- ❋ If we stand up for ourselves and are true to ourselves and say what we feel, others can understand us far better than when we maintain a false front.

A story and questions: Karin and the blackberries

Karin was 45 years old. She lived with her 70-year-old mother in a house with a large garden that they both enjoyed.

Karin had major surgery for breast cancer. Returning home after the operation was a happy moment: Karin was relieved and pleased to be out of hospital and able to rest in her own space and turn to her own recovery.

Her mother greeted her joyfully, but then immediately wanted to take her to the garden. The blackberries were ripe and 'needed' picking right away! She has been anxious about them and was so glad Karin was back in time to harvest them.

What do you think Karin felt at this moment?

Karin knows inside what she needs: she has an overwhelming desire to rest and to follow her own plans, not her mother's. She needs this far more than she will ever need the blackberries. But Karin also doesn't want to disappoint her mother.

Karin's mother's underlying need is no doubt less about future blackberry jam, and more about reassurance that there will be no change, that Karin is going to make sure the routines of the house and garden continue.

* What course of action, for Karin, is going to make it more likely that some care of her mother and the house and garden can continue long-term?
* If Karin picks the blackberries now, against her own instinct for what she needs, is she giving her mother a true message of reassurance or a false one?
* If Karin says 'no' to picking the blackberries, her mother will feel disappointed, but what else will she feel? What else might she learn?
* In Karin's situation, how would you reply?

Challenging our illusions

We all build illusions in circumstances where we don't want to accept the truth, or where there is a problem we don't think we can solve. Our minds try to suppress reality, usually unconsciously. Yet we do really know, inwardly and beyond doubt, that hopes and wishes are not the same as reality. And when we can bring illusions to consciousness for ourselves, we will know that ridding ourselves of them and accepting the truth is desirable and healthy. The capacity to recognise reality and to act accordingly is something we must all keep refreshing and practising anew.

We can see this process of dispelling illusion – of rejecting what is not true in reality or true to ourselves – as analogous to our immune system repeatedly checking what belongs to the body and what is alien, in order to keep restoring our health.

Where those around us are living inside illusion, we can help maintain their long-term health and our own by gently asserting our boundaries and the reality we see, and thus helping to dispel their illusion.

Disillusionment (with the disappointment this sometimes necessitates) rearranges the boundaries between people in ways that can be liberating and health-giving.

We can maintain our boundaries while finding empathy for ourselves and for others.

We can practise saying 'no' lovingly, each day.

An exercise: How to say 'no'

Return to the earlier exercise in this chapter when you tried to recall a situation in which you had felt 'no' but said 'yes'.

Imagine yourself into that situation again, and think about how you could have said a firm but loving 'no'. How would you phrase it?

Try saying the words out loud.

* How would that feel?
* How would it feel for those you are speaking to?
* How would it feel the next day?
* How would it feel many days later?

Saying 'no' when you need to will ultimately be a blessing for you and for others. It is you acknowledging yourself, your inner voice, the voice of your own heart. It is vital to self-love.

Tips: to help you say 'no'

* Try to predict 'no' situations in advance and ready yourself for them
* Prepare appropriate 'no' phrases that you would be comfortable using in different situations
* State your 'no' phrase clearly and keep eye contact with the other person
* Say 'no' without offering excuses – giving one simple reason is fine
* Don't waver: stick to your 'no'[43]

Learning to say 'no' in a way that feels comfortable is a significant step along the road to good health. If you are learning this skill as a result of an illness, you can see your illness as a signpost that has pointed the way back to yourself.

Focusing on what is essential to you

Many years ago, I went for a long walk with my father. He was 56, and had been diagnosed with a tumour. Memorably, he said to me: 'I want to focus on essentials now.'

Since then, I have had long talks with many people coming to terms with such an illness, and I've learned that this impulse is common in such circumstances. We have an innate desire to concentrate on important things, but that desire is often pushed aside or suppressed by other priorities. Illness can give us the chance to pursue what we most want, to be who we really are.

Steve Jobs, entrepreneur and co-founder of Apple Inc., gave a legendary talk to students at Stanford University when he was gravely ill. He talked about the importance of being fully yourself:

> Your time is limited, so don't waste it living someone else's life. Don't be trapped by dogma – which is living with the results of other people's thinking. Don't let the noise of others' opinions drown out your own inner voice. And most important, have the courage to follow your heart and intuition. They somehow already know what you truly want to become. Everything else is secondary.[44]

The feeling that you are truly pursuing your own path will make you more 'unassailable' in many respects. In my work I have been privileged to meet many people with serious illnesses who have come to concentrate on their inmost impulses, their true nature. In some this 'inner autonomy' had led them to such inner peace that they felt they had been cured even if they were to die of their illness.

Autonomy

When seriously ill, conductor Christoph Schlingensief described his priorities like this:

> I just want to retain my autonomy. I find it so important for patients to know they are autonomous, and not wholly governed by their doctor or their illness. All these things have to be put in their proper place since it is so easy to lose yourself in your illness.[45]

Autonomy during medical treatment

Many patients feel the need to reflect on how to change their life from the first onset of their illness. They often find it hard to get medical professionals to understand these inner imperatives, and feel that only their illness is perceived, not themselves as whole human beings. Then they face the challenge of standing up for themselves.

What do we do when our inner voice conflicts with doctors' proposals for our treatment, when they try to enforce recommendations as directives? (In passing we should mention that something is very wrong when 'ideal' guidelines, intended as orientation for patients, are increasingly seen as fixed rules they are obliged to follow!)

There are patients who have found the strength to communicate their needs and their experience clearly to their physician. Others follow their inner voice and seek out a different physician who is willing to fully engage with them.

When suffering from a life-threatening illness, quite particularly, it is very important that we cultivate gentle and loving regard for ourselves, and connect with people, including medical professionals, who affirm that regard and our own autonomy.

People who clearly perceive what they feel and can stand up for themselves are more positively involved in their treatment than those who simply do what they're told. This is self-evident. Such people, even if they are thought to be 'awkward' patients, often seem to have better outcomes.

As we know, the capacity to act autonomously is intimately connected with the body's ability to maintain its own boundaries. Autonomy right down to the cellular level is a key aspect of our health.

In studies involving several thousand patients, Ronald Grossarth-Maticek, formerly professor at Heidelberg University, established a clear connection between autonomy and prognosis.[46]

Aaron Antonovsky, the medical sociologist who first coined the term 'salutogenesis', studied the origins of health, rather than studying disease. He studied people who had lived through great stress but had survived it and continued to be healthy. He, too, came to the conclusion that it makes a vital difference whether people feel themselves to be victims or co-creators of what happens to them. According to Antonovsky, health is largely dependent on whether we experience the world we live in as comprehensible – whether we feel that we ourselves can affect what is happening, can shape it and perceive meaning in it.

For health, we need to be able to develop a 'sense of coherence', feeling ourselves to be part of a whole, meaningful context. Three parameters have a decisive effect on how we experience situations, and how our physical and emotional defensive forces are strengthened or weakened. Those three parameters are whether our circumstances feel:

1. comprehensible,
2. manageable,
3. meaningful.[47]

Inner resources

Remember that a tumour cell fails to assume the differentiating, autonomous developmental form normally present in the body. Its form and configuration is not pervaded by the otherwise normal law of self-structuring, and instead remains, in a sense, underdeveloped and embryonic in nature. We could see this as analogous to a situation in which we have lost our psychological sense of coherence and integration. Just as we can regain our autonomy and purpose as individuals, our body has the wisdom and potential to help an 'underdeveloped' tumour cell achieve healthy differentiation again, or to dissolve the cell.

Haematologist and oncologist Gerd Nagel, who himself overcame a practically incurable form of leukaemia, said the following:

> It seems to me that we have far, far greater inner curative powers than we realise, and that these can overcome illnesses such as cancer. The difficulty lies in knowing or discovering to what degree a particular patient standing before me has this potential. This isn't something we can generalise about, for orthodox medicine and medical practice are highly schematised. People always apply certain schemas. When it is a matter of drawing on a person's own resources in the healing process, their self-healing powers, we first have to discover these. And there lies the problem: discovering what potential each individual person has. ... It is certainly important to indicate early on that this inner resource exists, these curative forces exist, and that this is an opportunity to be used. But there is no guarantee, either, that what one might hope for in this regard will actually come about.

> I am fairly extreme in my views about this, but I feel that it is really a scandal that our health system concerns itself so little with the 'competent' patient. I think we should be shouting this from

the rooftops. Treatment is funded but, apart from rehabilitative medicine, no attention is given to things that nurture patient competency and put patients back in the context of ordinary life. I am sure that this form of consultation will have to find a place in the health systems of the future.[48]

If doctors understood health

Neurobiologist Gerald Hüther reported on the following experience, when he tried to teach future doctors about the human body's capacity for health and healing:

> I tried to offer a course of lectures for medical students at my university on 'Salutogenesis and self-healing'. The commission responsible for approving such courses asked for my patience. The problem was that the 'learning objectives' list for medical studies contains over a hundred objectives, from wound dressing to completing a death certificate, but makes no reference whatsoever to terms like 'salutogenesis', let alone 'self-healing'. The learning objectives for future doctors therefore do not include acquiring insight into what keeps a person healthy, nor the reorganisation processes at work in a body that is recovering from illness.

> In the minds of most doctors, clearly, including those who train our future doctors, is a firmly rooted conviction that people fall ill because something isn't functioning properly in their bodies, and that it is their task to discover this defect, repair it, and thus cure a patient of their disease. Those who think like this cannot, of course, get very far with the findings of research into salutogenesis and self-healing.[49]

All living systems, and thus every ecosystem or social system, every organism as bodily system, and not least out own nervous system, shape and form themselves, developing their respective structural and functional characteristics through ongoing adaptation of their particular subsystem relationships to the requirements of a continually changing outer world. ... If we understand this, then it is also self-evident that no one can cure another person, but that every cure is an expression of the same self-organising process that is now at work in more favourable conditions, which enable it to 'heal' again.

The highest art of medicine involves accompanying this self-healing process as competently as possible, with the help of all the procedures and tools of medical science and medical technology. This will be the key task of a medicine of the future.[50]

I decide what I wish, and which path I take

We can decide which path to follow when we have an idea or a picture of a goal. We won't set out on the journey without some such vision. It is clear that the better delineated this inner vision is, the stronger a resource it offers on our path. It is important for patients, therefore, to keep creating their own vivid pictures and visions of health.

Without this belief, without this vision that health is possible regardless of doctors' opinions and medical remedies, very few patients will embark on the healing journey. In order to heal, patients need to formulate a clear resolve: 'I wish to be healthy! I will strengthen my health.'

But to turn this resolve into practical action is a further step, one in which we must say something like, 'I will do what I feel, believe and know will help me recover.'

An exercise: I will do what makes me healthy

This exercise comes from Dr. Carl Simonton. Say this sentence out loud:

'I have decided to do what I feel, believe and know will help me recover.'

Notice all the complexities of how you feel as you say it.

How much conviction or strength do you feel as you say it? How much hesitation or doubt?

Some people feel an insuperable obstacle to saying this sentence. This may indicate that at present they are not yet in a place where they can experience themselves as co-creators of their own lives, able to take things into their own hands.

Acknowledging this is helpful. It can tell you what steps you need to take.

A question: positive changes

Since you fell ill, have there been changes in and around you for which you feel grateful?

This may seem an odd, or even an offensive, question. Illness brings many negative changes, many negative feelings: fear, shock, doubt, anger, disappointment, pain and loss. How, then, can there be any room for positive experiences?

I have found that many of my patients do in fact accord real value to their time of illness and credit it with many positive feelings and realisations. I have also found that many patients feel almost ashamed to recognise and express the positive benefits of their illness. Perhaps doing so would make others think they had chosen their illness or were 'indulging' in it. They have kept such things concealed, because it has been too awkward to acknowledge and express them.

But if patient groups talk together, they find their positive experiences are almost invariably shared by others.

If you feel able, perhaps write down some of the changes you feel grateful for, which you have noticed since being ill.

In my seminar groups for patients, many of the changes people describe have turned out to be common to all there. There may be positive changes in their experience of time, in being more aware of themselves, in learning to say no when they need to. Do you recognise any of these statements?

- ❋ 'I suddenly had time for myself again. Time to think and feel.'
- ❋ 'I let go of my usual schedule, and had so much time in which to just be.'
- ❋ 'I feel more awake.'
- ❋ 'I am more aware of my own limits.'
- ❋ 'I live more consciously.'
- ❋ 'I see clearly what is truly important to me.'
- ❋ 'I have been thinking about the meaning of my life.'
- ❋ 'My relationships with others have become full of meaning.'
- ❋ 'I have let go of others' expectations and demands.'

❋ 'I have allowed myself to feel again. I don't suppress my feelings any more or dismiss them – they have become too insistent for that.'

❋ 'I started going for a walk every day.'

❋ 'I met up with an old friend I had wanted to see for ages.'

❋ 'I have joined a choir and started singing again.'

❋ 'I gave up certain tasks I found very difficult. I would never have dreamed of stopping before I fell ill; now I have let them go.'

❋ 'I have learned to ask for help.'

❋ 'I no longer feel I have to prove myself.'

❋ 'I can distinguish what is essential.'

❋ 'I feel more contact and closeness with nature, and cycles of life and death.'

❋ 'I feel more gratitude and love.'

Finding meaning

Many patients experience great changes at an inner level: not in their bodily health, not as a result of surgery or treatment, but in their essential being. Many say they value life more. They have learned to be more present in the moment.

Most patients feel more in touch with themselves.

This insight can open a door to finding meaning in illness. People who find meaning in what happens to them gain much more strength to cope with it. Trauma research has shown that if we can find meaning in the bad things that happen to us, we are more likely to return to strength.

Illness can be seen as an invitation to reflect lovingly on how to be the person you are and wish to be.

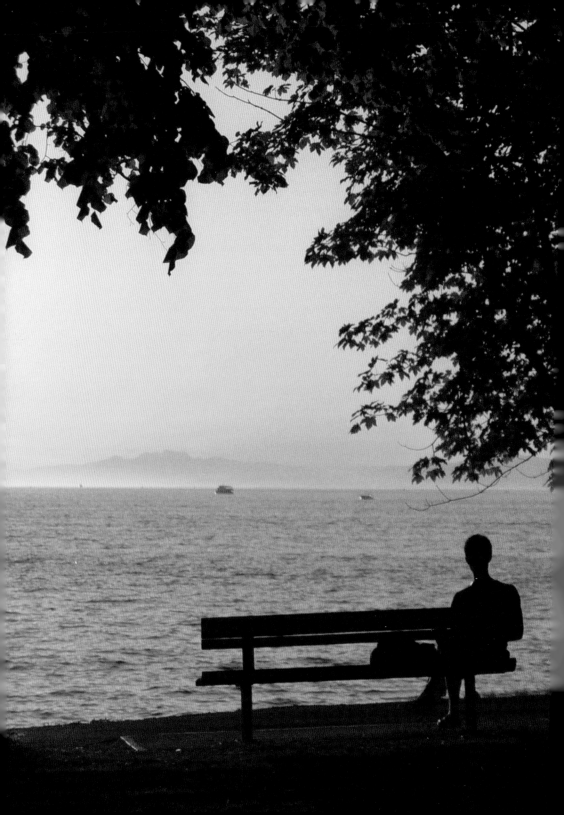

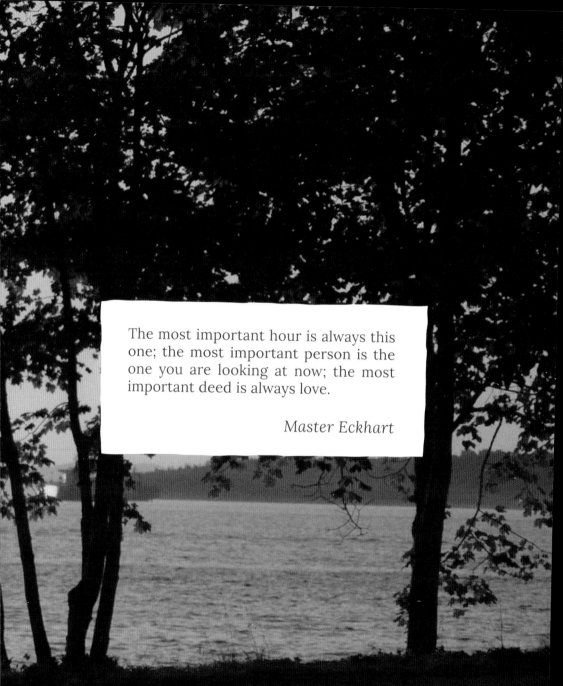

The most important hour is always this one; the most important person is the one you are looking at now; the most important deed is always love.

Master Eckhart

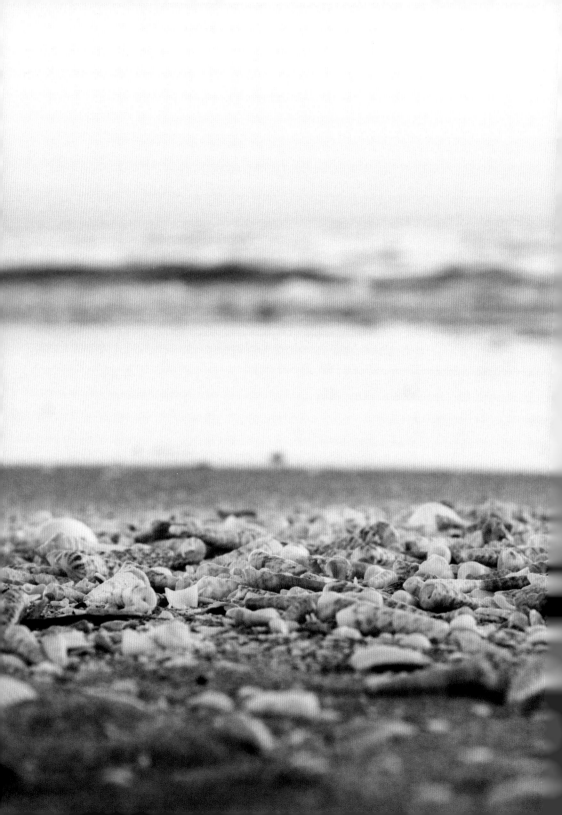

Managing Questions of Fault and Blame

Finding the cause

If you stand on the beach in the morning you can tell how stormy it was last night by the amount of flotsam and jetsam. The appearance of the beach allows us to tell what the sea was like in the night.

Some people regard an illness as a symptom, the expression of an underlying cause.

Imagine that the oil gauge in your car shows the oil is very low. The 'symptom' could be fixed by forcing the oil indicator up by hand to point to 'normal' again. But that won't fix the cause of the low indicator.

It is important to distinguish between cause and symptom. It would be pointless to keep pumping up a flat tyre if there's a nail sticking in it. The cause of the flat tyre has to be recognised and remedied.

The mental picture we create of an illness matters. For example, is a tumour a cause of illness, or a symptom of a more long-standing process? If we imagine that the tumour is the sole cause of the problem, and not the symptom of a process, we might well think that getting rid of it will cure the cancer. Surgeons often suggest this to patients.

One of my patients talked about this. He didn't feel the surgeon's point of view reflected his experience of illness. His sense was that the illness was part of him, about him and belonged to him. The surgeon could help, he thought, but after the surgery there would still be work for him to do himself.

Who is the protagonist of the illness?

For some patients, the illness and its symptoms are a challenge that they feel is fundamentally connected with their way of living and being. Equally, there are people who cannot find any explanation for their illness in their own lives.

Perhaps such questioning is pointless. Many patients are not interested in whether a tumour is a symptom or cause. The just want to get rid of it.

But the challenge of a severe illness presents us with two goals simultaneously: one is treatment of the particular condition. The other is strengthening our underlying health. In the case of cancer this means strengthening the organising power at work in our body so that cell division and cellular reorganisation happens in a healthy way from then on. Removal of the tumour does not automatically lead to restoration of the healthy reorganising capacity.

Many patients who face the challenge of a severe illness for the first time in their lives find it very hard to grasp that they themselves can make a difference to their situation. The situation is new and alien, and they will only do what doctors tell them to. Some patients change this perspective once they have been struggling for some time with their illness and have acquired experience. It can take a long time for an ill person to feel that they are in fact the chief protagonist of their illness story, the agent of their own recovery.

Blaming oneself

But the question then arises: if a severe illness is related to my way of life, if its progress is something I could have influenced, if I am not just a victim but also a co-creator, then surely I am to blame for my illness?

This thought can make illness even more unbearable for many patients.

People handle the question of the cause of their illness in very different ways. Some forbid themselves from asking it but others pay great attention to discovering where, how and when something in their life fell out of balance.

The dominant view among health professionals working in oncology is that it is bad when patients blame themselves for their illness. But unfortunately this view can lead to a complete separation in the way we all consider illness and the patient's life and circumstances.

This separation of illness and the patient's life unburdens the patient. The patient bears no responsibility for the illness. But at the same time, patients are disempowered. If the patient is not really involved in becoming ill, then the patient also has little role in the cure.

Of course, there should never be any blame involved. But I doubt whether we get closer to life's realities by completely avoiding the question of how we may have played a part in our own illnesses.

Different understandings of responsibility

In relation to grave illnesses, the issue of blame needs to be handled very sensitively. Some oncologists regard cancer patients as dealing with three traumas:

1. The shock of diagnosis – and my patients always report that the time, place and manner of communication makes a big difference.
2. The trauma of surgery.
3. The impact of follow-up treatment.

Someone already dealing with this threefold trauma should not also have to deal with issues of guilt or blame.

Yet we also need to be able to connect the biochemical processes of pathology to life circumstances, interiority and our development as human beings.

Understanding what responsibility means

Patients think about causal connections and blame very differently. Some see their illness as personal failure. Some even see it as punishment. Yet there are others who can entertain the idea that they might need to make changes without resorting to chastising themselves. These patients can understand that there may be connections between life and illness without framing those connections in moral terms.

Those who blame themselves can get stuck, unable to let go of the past. Those who can consider the connections without getting mired in accusation can turn to the future. The connections empower and invigorate them to embark on a new course.

It seems to me that the issue of blame or fault is intimately related to each person's life experiences and convictions. In some it leads to paralysis, despair and humiliation while for others it can open the way to inner clarity and new impetus.

The limits of finding fault

I have a role in shaping my own life and my own circumstances. But that doesn't mean that the many effects of each of my actions can easily be described as my 'fault'.

Often we are unaware of the consequences of our actions at the moment we act. There are many effects of any action, and we can never weigh them all beforehand. No one has total choice; all of our choices are constrained and are made in situations of limited knowledge. We can never take full responsibility for outcomes, but nor is it helpful to avoid recognising the connections between the outcomes and our actions and choices. Our minds cannot always encompass all the repercussions of our own conduct, but as we recognise the repercussions slowly over time, we can adjust, re-tune and improve things in a gradual process to develop a healthier life.

Perfectionism

What kind of view of the human being has led us to our modern culture of blame and accusation? Perhaps we are governed, among other things, by perfectionism, by the view that we could and should get everything right if we just tried harder. This mode of thought is intrinsically alien to life and development. Perhaps we believe we ought to control every aspect of ourselves and our bodies, but as soon as we step back and look at such an assumption, we can see we would not be human if we did.

The small and interior choices I make daily become large and exterior effects over time. This wisdom is found in the Talmud:

> Attend to your thoughts for they become words.
> Attend to your words for they become actions.
> Attend to your actions for they become habits.
> Attend to your habits for they become your character.
> Attend to your character for it becomes your destiny.

Yet I am far from the sole force shaping my life.

A study of the factors involved in developing cancer

Denmark records the genetic data of all its citizens. This means the Danes have an excellent database for genetic studies. One of these studies looked at a thousand children who were adopted at birth to see whether their chance of contracting cancer was affected if one of their genetic parents had died of cancer before the age of 50. The finding was 0 per cent increase in cancer rates in these children. However, if an *adoptive* parent died of cancer before the age of 50, the incidence of cancer in their adopted children increased fivefold.[51] This study suggests that life circumstances are a more decisive factor in our risk of cancer than genetics. Does this mean that the adopted children who contract cancer are to blame for contracting it? Of course not. Does it mean that we might all be able to have some effect on our own chance of developing cancer? Quite possibly.

Acting in good faith

We often develop by learning, painfully, from our mistakes. But blame is probably not appropriate if we made mistakes when acting in good faith, and with the best knowledge we had at the time.

Many patients look back and see that they have made choices against their own knowledge, that they have taxed themselves too severely, that they have accepted levels of stress in their lives that they knew were excessive.

To access untapped developmental potential in ourselves we need to be able to examine our own past, and be empowered to make decisions that will change the future.

Perceiving without judgement

We are all different. While many patients with a serious illness decide it is up to them to make changes and lead a healthier life, others very much want everything to go back to the way it was before.

It seems necessary to me to develop a perspective on illness that is without judgement or accusation. Only then can we let go of reproach and of self-reproach.

Self-knowledge need not automatically lead to putting oneself in the dock. There are other ways of relating to our past than to set ourselves up as our own judge and prosecutor. Condemnation does not align with the idea that we are always developing.

We live according to our capacities

For many patients, the acknowledgment that something is out of balance in their lives becomes an impulse or invitation to create new equilibrium. Dr Hans Werner, co-founder of the Eschelbronn Clinic, said that he would like to exchange the concept of blame for that of 'capacity'. This seems right to me.

We live according to our current capacities, and according to our current awareness. We can only shape our lives from our present position and understanding.

But we can all learn and mature. We can create change. We have opportunities throughout life to learn and gain new experience. Illness can be a particularly powerful opportunity.

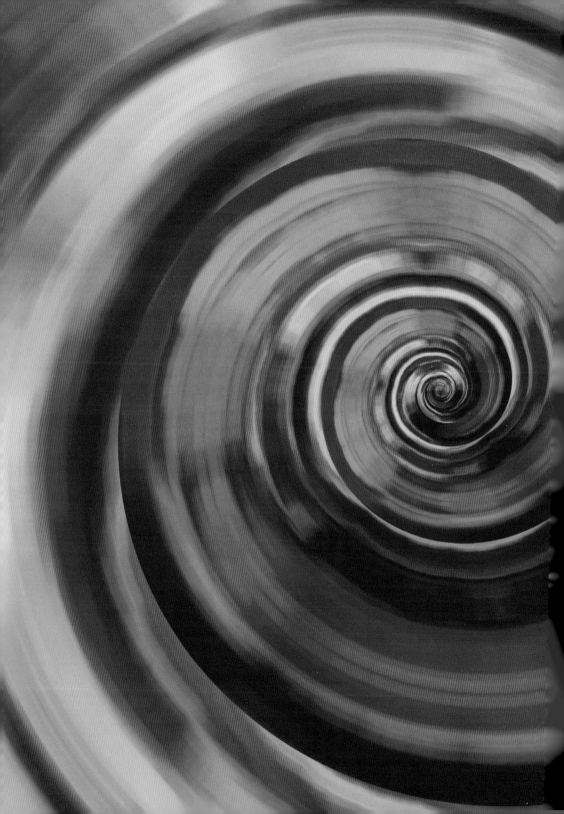

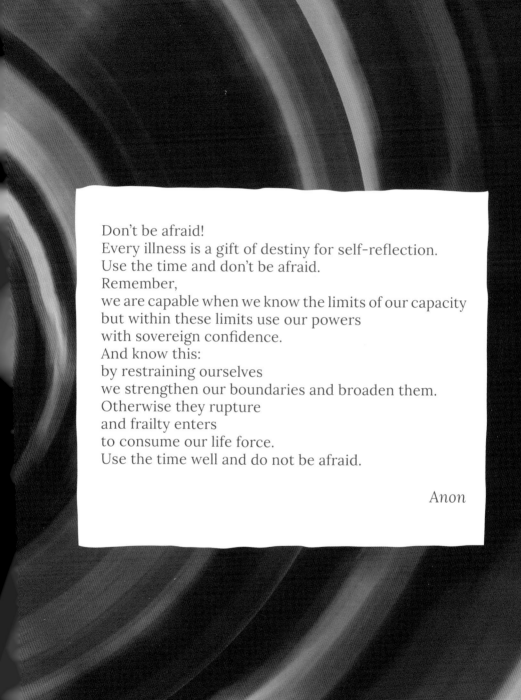

Don't be afraid!
Every illness is a gift of destiny for self-reflection.
Use the time and don't be afraid.
Remember,
we are capable when we know the limits of our capacity
but within these limits use our powers
with sovereign confidence.
And know this:
by restraining ourselves
we strengthen our boundaries and broaden them.
Otherwise they rupture
and frailty enters
to consume our life force.
Use the time well and do not be afraid.

Anon

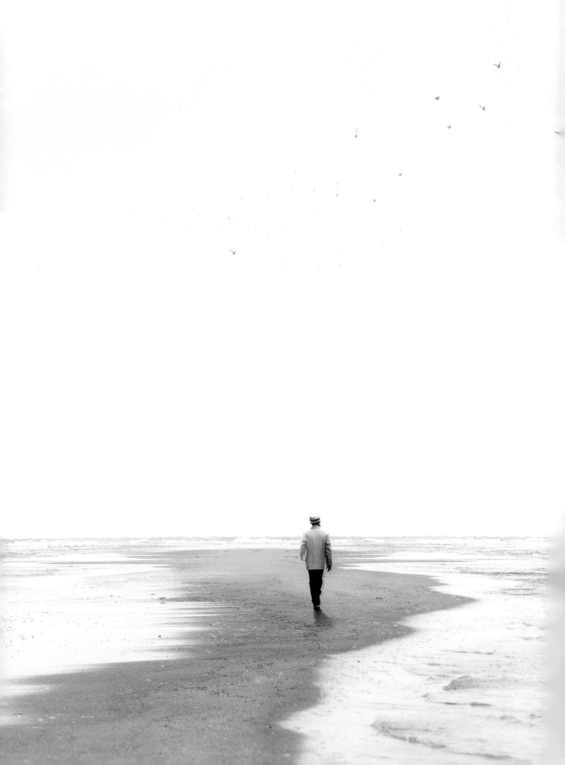

Dealing with Anxiety

Anxiety can be enabling or disabling

In a situation of acute crisis, fear and anxiety can save my life, lending me the strength to take decisive action.

On the other hand, chronic and ongoing anxiety can paralyse me, and prevent me having full presence of mind in the moment. It is this kind of fear or anxiety I need to address. Addressing it does not mean suppressing or ignoring it, but facing up to it, looking directly at it as anxiety.

Usually we flee fear, try to shake it off or distract ourselves. But if the same thoughts keep surfacing all the time, depriving us of sleep or affecting our quality of life, we will need to look for other ways of dealing with them, and aim for long-term solutions.

One of my patients said that he was plagued by anxiety at night, so he always read a book. If he wasn't reading he would compulsively worry about the future: fear-inducing pictures would rise up in his mind.

Diversionary tactics of this kind can be useful in the moment. But they are not dealing with the underlying cause of the anxiety.

An exercise: observing anxiety

The first step in tackling anxiety is learning to observe our own thoughts. Rather than being carried along by thoughts, step back and watch them.

Some of our thoughts are perceptions of external reality, some will be our own interpretations, judgements and attempts to create meaning. These will be jumbled up together.

Notice whether you have thoughts that invoke trust and confidence along with thoughts that inspire fear and anxiety.

Our thoughts are never a pure stream of perception of the outside world. They always contain our own perspective, and this means distortions can occur.

See whether you can distinguish between perceptions of reality and your own connections, interpretations and assumptions.

By using the power of our intentionally governed attention – our 'I' – we can observe our own processes of integration and absorption. We can start to distinguish between what is certain and real, and what are our own fears and distortions taking over.

When fearful thoughts surface, such as 'I can't go on' or 'Everything's hopeless' or 'I'm alone', first try to observe them.

Do they come with mental pictures, even with a whole storyline like a film?

What stories are you telling yourself about what is happening and what might happen?

Do these mental pictures and stories feel hypothetical, or have they started to feel like actual reality, already unfolding?

This practice of watching your own anxious thoughts and then distinguishing between what you are seeing in the world and what you are mentally creating can in itself start to tackle anxiety.

By consciously observing our feelings and thoughts, we shift from being helplessly fearful into the more dispassionate mode of investigator.

Try, too, writing down your anxiety-inducing thoughts. Perhaps keep a specific journal only for this purpose. Writing thoughts, like observing them, helps us separate from them. They feel like they are outside us rather than inside. We can then more easily see that they are not totalising facts, but interpretations and possibilities and stories about an unknowable future. By externalising on the page, we may feel less controlled by them.

When we engage our minds to consciously reflect on our anxious predictions, we can often recognise that they are only one aspect of the many possibilities life holds.

How to consider a prognosis

Many patients with serious illness feel understandable fear and anxiety about the prognosis they have been given by their doctors. The words doctors have used when explaining how serious the illness is and to predict the chances of recovery can become obsessive thoughts. Yet it is almost impossible for medical professionals to offer an accurate prognosis in any particular case. This is one of those situations when the distinction between what is actual reality and what are our thoughts and interpretations is most helpful, and most easily lost. Doctors' words tend to have great weight with our emotions, but our healthy common sense ought to be very wary of any general prognosis applied to us as a specific individual.

For all their training and experience, doctors are not clairvoyant. They, like all of us, cannot see the future. As a statistician patient of mine put it:

a prognosis is a statistical summary of very specific circumstances and therefore not directly applicable to a particular individual.

Prognoses are based on the percentage of past patients who have recovered from an illness, but they cannot tell any individual how ill their own body is or what its power of recovery might be. For people who completely recover from an illness, the percentage was irrelevant: they were not 30 per cent ill, they were ill and are now well.

In 1995, at the invitation of Deutsche Krebshilfe (German Cancer Aid Society), a group of doctors from various countries met in Heidelberg to study people who, in the view of medicine, had no chance of recovery but who recovered despite this prognosis. By the end of their conference the doctors had come to the view that a word should be removed from medical vocabulary: incurable. Reflecting on the experience of meeting so many cured incurables, Professor Walter M. Gallmeier said:

> If someone does not see what is there in front of them, which anyone can see, or refuses to see it because it is currently inexplicable, they are no longer being truly scientific. Scientifically oriented doctors are also allowed to be astonished and pose questions.

'There are more things in heaven and earth ... than are dreamt of in your philosophy,' says Shakespeare's Hamlet. Despite our inability to explain seemingly 'miraculous' recoveries, we must still acknowledge that they happen. In doing so we can respect the fact that there are powerful healing forces within us.

In a serious illness, no one can predict the eventual outcome. There are general experiences that point to possible tendencies, but no individual is pre-programmed. We know that a disease can be life-threatening, but we also know that recovery is possible.

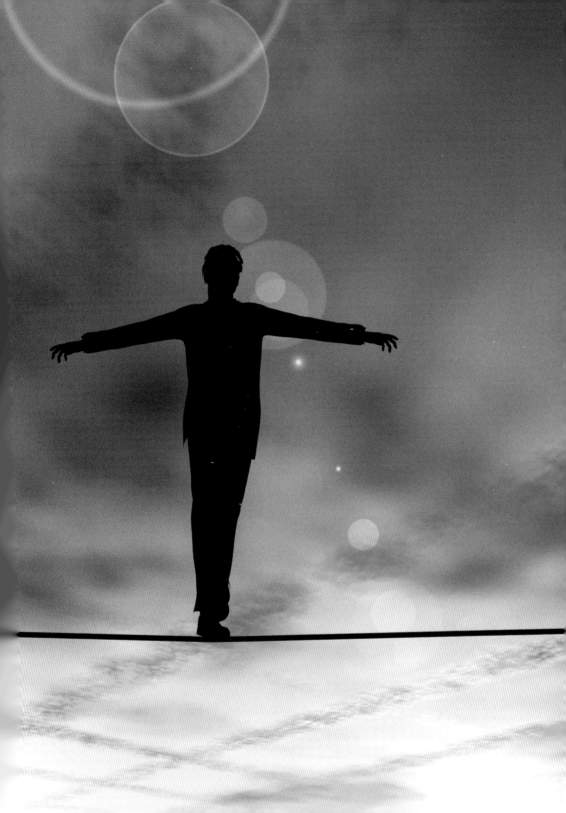

The tightrope walker

Imagine the mental state of the tightrope walker. The tightrope walker is very calm. All they need to do is walk steadily forwards. The tightrope walker concentrates on putting one foot in front of the other and maintaining forward motion. If they focus instead on the emptiness beneath, they may well fall.

In times of fear and uncertainty, as long as we have no better information, it can help to purposely develop desirable scenarios in our own minds. Picture things turning out well. If we haven't considered all the desirable outcomes, our minds may only focus on negative possibilities.

Uncertainty is not the problem, but rather the thoughts that rise in us because of it. Uncertainty gives us an opportunity to develop pictures of a desirable outcome.

It is not helpful or realistic to block out all our worries, to discount our feelings or our experience. Our worries are there for a reason. They encourage us to take necessary precautions and prepare for possible difficulties. But they are not the whole story or the only likely outcome.

The power of trust

When faced with uncertainty, we often respond by trying to find as much information as possible. In the age of the internet, information can seem infinite: we feel the certainty we are seeking must be hiding there somewhere. Information is indeed important, and sometimes finding out more will solve the problem. Sometimes there is an answer and we can discover it and the uncertainty is gone. But often this isn't the case.

There is no final answer and no matter how long we search the uncertainty remains. When information can't help resolve things for us, we have to rely instead on the power of trust.

It is possible to create an inner certainty even when information cannot provide outside certainty for us. Many patients find that they have a place of safety inside themselves where they are confident in the future. Not that they can be confident of any particular outcomes, but they are quietly certain that they can withstand what might come, they trust that they will be accorded spiritual protection. I would describe this as a 'spiritual cloak'.

How can we find our way to this inner confidence?

Many people find succour from certain prayers that they speak, or rituals they practise, or from reading particular texts.

An exercise: strengthening tranquillity

Remember Rudolf Steiner's meditative verse:

Tranquillity I bear within.
I bear within myself
the forces that strengthen me.
I fill myself
with their warmth,
Now I fill myself
with my own will's resolve,
and I feel tranquillity
pouring through my being.
When, by my steadfast striving,
I become strong
to find within
the source of strength,
the strength of tranquillity.

Neurologist Dr. Christian Schopper suggests a threefold approach to this meditation. If you have the opportunity, try this together with someone else or in a group, or you can also do it on your own.

1. Read the text aloud twice to yourself or to another person. While you are reading, try to grasp what the words are saying.
2. Then read the text aloud twice just listening to its melody without trying to grasp its content.
3. As a third step, read the text aloud twice and try to *absorb* it. Sense what inward effect it has on you.

Anxiety as a helpful indicator

It may be that anxious thoughts are telling us we are not yet properly prepared for something, or that some inner or outer change is needed. If we then ignore these fears, and do not make the necessary preparations or changes, the anxiety will grow until we acknowledge and attend to it. We can understand anxiety and fear as signposts, pointing our attention to something important.

In the chapter titled 'Death as Life's Assistant' we met three walkers going up into the Swiss Alps in October. One was preparing only for summery weather, one only for wintery weather, and the third was preparing for both possibilities. Most people find the third option the least anxious one.

Can you bring this third way of thinking to your illness, to the tests and procedures you will undergo? Can you manage anxiety by working and hoping for the best outcome but being prepared for a worse one?

Focus on getting positive results but at the same time consider how to deal with a less positive outcome, and where you would turn for help and advice. Anxiety is a signpost, pointing us in the direction of finding help, of knowing where our support will be if we should need it.

Underneath everything else, this means being prepared both to live and to die. If you are not prepared, anxiety may be prompting you to think harder about either or both of these possibilities. Underneath, your anxiety may be asking you: do you wish to be healthy, and if so why? What is your purpose in being alive here on earth? Or it might be asking you: how might you prepare for dying and death? If you were to leave this plane of existence, what inner state would you like to be in when you do so?

This double stance of expecting the best but being prepared for things to take a different course helps ensure that anxiety does not take hold. We acknowledge and face our anxiety, using it as a signpost, rather than being overwhelmed by it.

A story: I am not afraid of my illness

An oncologist who is a friend of mine told me about a patient who had advanced and inoperable breast cancer. She didn't want to have chemotherapy; she was sure this would do her more harm than good. My friend therefore proposed other forms of treatment for her.

The unusual thing about this patient was that she said she knew *why* she had fallen ill, and also that she was not afraid of her illness. 'For many years,' she told him, 'I always tried to please my husband. But this wasn't good for me, so I have stopped all that now. I know that my illness isn't my enemy, and I am not afraid. I know that I have been given no burden greater than my power to bear it.'

For this woman, illness was not a nasty threat, it was a message about her life in a form she couldn't ignore.

This patient had a deep unshakeable trust in her safety. She recovered, and ten years later was still well.

Feeling safe in insecurity

Pablo Picasso once said, 'I do not seek, I find.'[52] He is also said to have uttered these words:

> Seeking is when you start from old things and rediscover what you already know. Finding is something entirely new, new and in motion. All paths are open and what you will discover is unknown. It is a risk, a sacred adventure. The uncertainty of such ventures can only be taken on by those who feel safe in insecurity, who allow ourselves to be led into the leaderless dark and there give themselves to an invisible star, who let themselves be drawn by the goal rather than narrowing and defining the goal themselves, as humans so often do. Openness to new experience, to every new occurrence both inside and outside us, is the key trait of modern human beings, who despite all the fear of letting go, can find themselves sustained by the grace of new, unfolding possibilities.

Tips: dealing with anxiety

When anxious thoughts arise, here are some practical things to try:

- At moments of anxiety first try breathing deeply.
- A patient told me that what helped her was accepting the anxiety rather than trying to suppress it or push it away. The fear of imminent anxiety was often worse for her than the anxiety itself. Since she had allowed herself to have anxiety, acknowledging and accepting it by 'going into it' and looking at it, she had found herself much better able to deal with it.
- Some people have poems, verses or mediations that they can recite at such moments.
- Many turn to prayer, and find this calms them.
- Another patient was having trouble falling asleep due to anxiety late at night. She took up a practice of looking back each evening on the past day to identify what she felt grateful for. Then she fell asleep with this sense of gratitude.
- Call to mind seemingly hopeless situations in your past. How did you get through them and survive? Many people say that they feel they received help and support precisely at their moments of greatest despair.

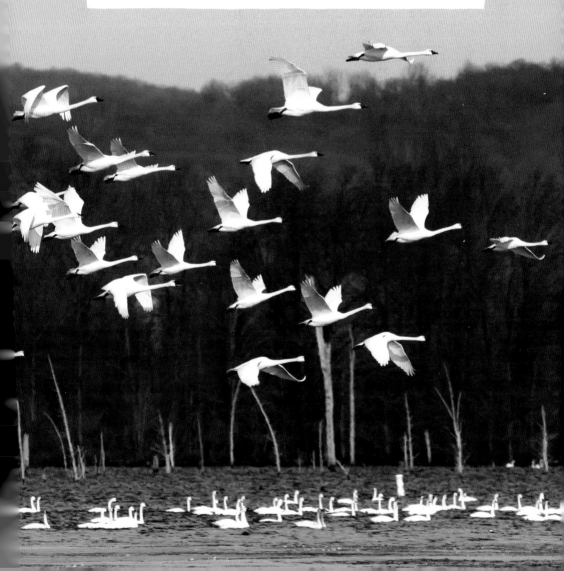

The moment you trust, you will know how to live.

Johann Wolfgang von Goethe

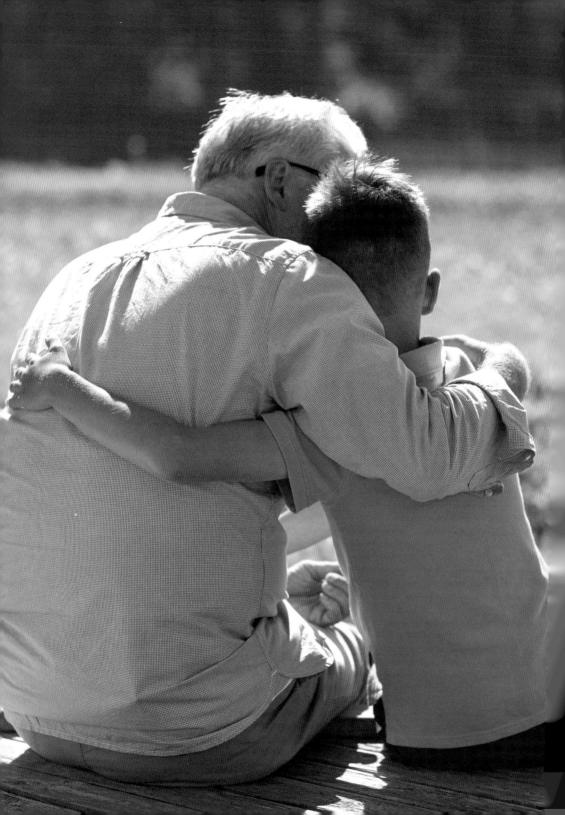

Trusting

What affects our mood; what our mood affects

How we are feeling, our mood, has an impact on our body. A doctor I know put it this way: 'Depression is not made of air. If we suffer from depression for a long time, this affects the body too.' The effects of anxiety on the body and brain have become apparent through recent developments in brain scanning.

But how does our mood come about? The spontaneous answer would be that it is due to what we experience, see and hear. Doubtless this is one side of the coin, but the other is our inner nature and how our experiences affect it: our inner state.

People do not all react in the same way or respond with the same feelings to events. Each of us has our own inner state and ways of responding, and this interiority plays a key role in the mood that arises in us in response to circumstances.

We can say that particular individuals have a generally more negative or more positive outlook and mood.

How can we develop the underlying mood in ourselves that we would wish to have? This is a challenge, especially when we face a serious illness.

But we can say that a positive mood will be influenced by the degree to which we have developed trust in our lives.

Finding joy

It does not have to be so difficult to rediscover joy in life. Going for a walk can bring great joy. It is wonderful to feel lovingly connected with something. We all have within us the capacity to be lovingly connected in some way.

The word 'connection' refers us back to the threefold sense of connection described at the beginning of this book: connection to ourselves, to others and to God or the universe. Loving connection is perhaps easiest with others. My relationship with myself is also vital to my health and mood.

And the third relationship of existential importance for me is with the invisible realm, God, the spiritual, or the universe. This is perhaps the most easily neglected of the three relationships, but it is crucial for trust. Given all the uncertainty we live with, a connection with spiritual benevolence is indeed something to wish for. We may find that there are moments in daily life when we sense broader powers sustaining us. Have you had any quiet inklings of this help, of the possibility of receiving it?

Trust

Trust is allowing one's mind to rest upon something. Trust is believing in something. It is always better to believe in something than not to believe in anything. Of course it is good to challenge our beliefs and see if they stand the test of time. But as long as I am still searching for a belief that stands this test, it is better to believe in something that can help me, even if this is not what I ultimately come to believe.

Dr Carl Simonton

Questions: believing in yourself

Do you feel that you believe in yourself?

Trust and belief in oneself is easily lost, especially in times of trouble.

If someone has lost trust in themselves, how can they re-establish it?

Look back on your life and your wealth of experience. Find the times when you knew you could trust yourself.

Take reassurance from this history. You are capable in so many ways.

Trust in others

While we can strengthen trust in ourselves, there are also limits to our abilities and our strength. Sometimes we reach the end of our tether. At these times, it's important to ask others for help – to trust in others as well as in ourselves.

Many people say they have been badly disappointed in life and can no longer trust anyone. That is a very sad state of affairs.

None of us can cope with life entirely alone. From birth onwards we receive support and help in all kinds of ways and from many different sides, though we may often be unaware of it. Where we do see it, it is good to acknowledge and value the support and help around us.

A guardian angel

Can you think of a situation in your life when things might have gone awry but didn't – a feeling you were kept safe? At such moments the barrier between the earthly world and the world of spirit vanishes. Then we feel that the idea of two separate worlds is misleading: the realm 'beyond' can also be experienced as being here, on earth and within us. We do not need to maintain this insistence on separation. We can assent to our heartfelt experience of connection with other realms, with, say, a 'guardian angel' who stands by us.

Recovery through trust

Cultivating trust in ourselves, in fellow human beings and in the heavenly realm or the universe means we can move forward with strength and tranquillity, even in the face of great difficulty. This can only enhance our powers of recovery.

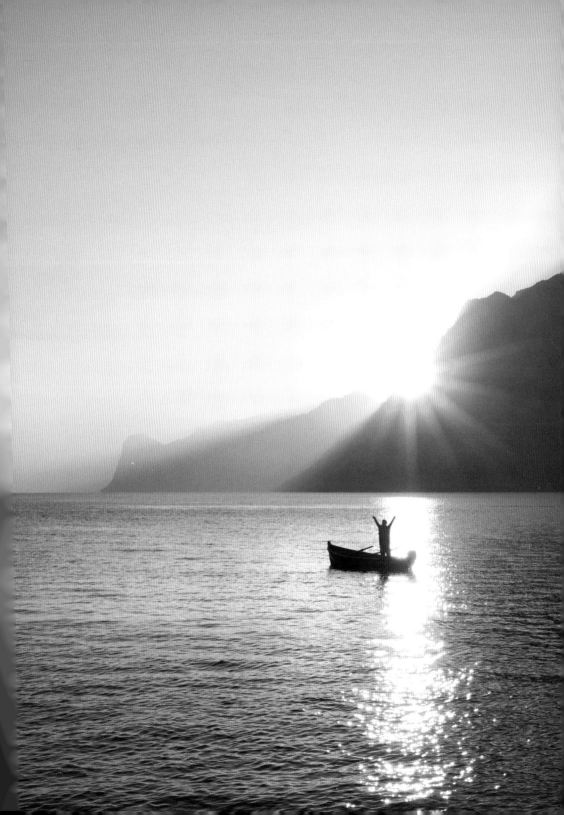

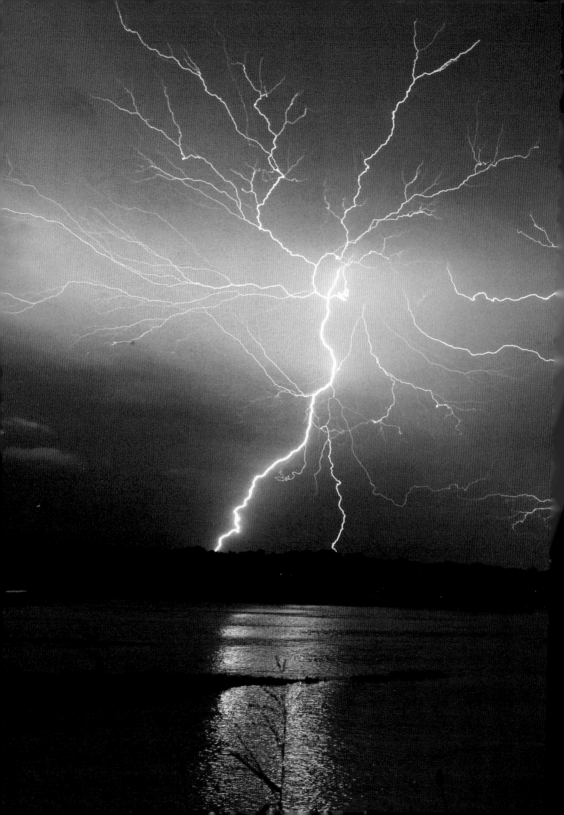

Cease doubting, picking all asunder
which makes the best things fall apart;
despite this world maintain your wonder
and faith in life with all your heart.

And heart, if you would find your health again,
be wholesome yourself, be true and pure.
All that we read in others and the world
is only our own reflection, you can be sure.

Theodor Fontane

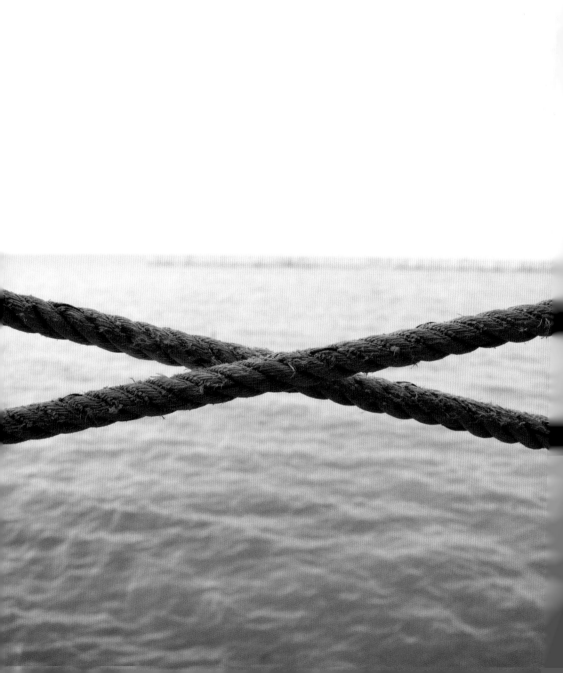

Handling Our Resentment, Anger and Hate

When we are stuck in the past

Positivity, tranquillity, love, authenticity, trust – all these qualities of recovery that we have been discussing are hard to achieve if we cannot make peace with ourselves, with others, with our situation, with destiny. What do we do if quite different feelings insist on surfacing?

We are all very different in how we relate to the past, the present and the future. Some people cling to the past, mourning the 'good old days'. Some people live in the past because they cannot let go of something that happened to them, something that was never resolved or integrated. Perhaps someone did something terrible to them, and they cannot understand why. Or they themselves may have done something they cannot forgive in themselves.

Sometimes feelings are so strong that resentment, anger or hatred bind us firmly to the past, and enormously restrict our ability to live in the present.

When we get stuck in resentment, rage or hate, our attention is no longer focused on ourselves. Our thoughts are 'away from home', sometimes even tumultuous – we are in a state in which we can no longer think clearly.

But if we can open ourselves up for help and support, we can deal with our own destructive forces. We can resolve and heal emotional dynamics that otherwise weaken and injure us.

Forgiveness and integration

First and foremost, we need to learn to forgive. But forgiveness doesn't mean a problem is instantly resolved. We have to mentally process and integrate the events that led to our resentment or anger. If I 'merely' forgive, outwardly and on the surface, but do not work through a process of assimilation, no real resolution has happened, and the issue will continue to live and ferment inside. While suppressing things and getting on with life can be a matter of survival in the short term, in the long term other solutions are needed.

People often say to each other that they should leave the past behind, and let go of grievances. But how do we actually do this?

We can't solve everything on our own: if there is an issue from the past that keeps making itself present in your feelings, seek help and support.

It is also worth looking forward and asking ourselves how to avoid taking on the same kinds of emotional burdens in the future. Are there patterns in your emotional struggles? Are there patterns in your difficult relationships? It is well worth taking time to reflect on such questions.

Integrating traumatic events

How do we psychologically integrate or assimilate traumatic events so that they are stitched into the past rather than constantly recurring in our minds in the present?

The first step is to name what happened: what was done, what was said. We cannot 'move on' until we can state clearly what our experience has been. Stating what happened involves recognising the difference between our perceptions and our analysis or interpretation of our perceptions. We need to try to strip away our analysis and state what happened as though a camera had recorded it – as though we are the camera, just observing and recording.

This is a good start to dealing with our past.

The next step is to bring to awareness the feelings these experiences spontaneously elicited in you at the time, and to be able to put a name on those feelings.

Once you can name your feelings at the time, perhaps you can recognise the fundamental needs in you that were overridden or violated. Try to name these too.[53]

Throughout this process it helps to have support from someone objective, who is not part of your everyday life, and who has training in guiding people through such emotional processing. There are outstanding trauma therapists practising today who have the 'tools' to transform deep-seated events and occurrences that go on rumbling and hurting us. Anyone who has suffered with deep emotional hurt or confusion would benefit from this professional help.

Before we get help we need to recognise that we don't have to solve everything alone. Rather, we can know that help is available, and we can allow ourselves to accept it.

Shifting our ongoing resentment and blame

How does resentment continue to live in us? What does the emotion feed upon? The usual way is we look for someone to blame – for doing, or not doing something, or perhaps many things. This was awful of them! They should be ashamed! They hurt me so much! That's why I feel resentment: because this person did this, or didn't do what they should have done.

Each time I remind myself vividly of the situation that led to my resentment, I am feeding it. Each time I ask myself 'How could they do such a thing?' Or think it all through again and come to the conclusion 'They should really never have done it!', I am clinging to these pictures of the wrong and fanning the flames of my anger.

How can we dry up this seemingly endless source of food for our resentment?

One way might be to allow ourselves to step out of the old picture – in other words we could try not pinning the person we blame or ourselves to the fixed point of a flaw or wrongdoing, but instead recognise that we are all on a journey of self-development, we are all constantly changing.

We all make mistakes. We can all learn and grow throughout our lives. When we last made a mistake, did we intend to? Usually this is not the case.

Our inner capacities or inadequacies are not as visible as a physical disability. Imagine if you had both arms in plaster after an accident: if a visitor came to greet you and shake you by the hand, you wouldn't be able to respond as usual, but the visitor will immediately understand why. No one would think you were impolite, no one would blame you. Psychologically, we are all wearing a number of invisible plaster casts. We all have blind spots, or ideas that need revision, or limitations that are still growing, or troubles we can't at present get beyond. There are places in the psyche where we make errors, knowingly or unknowingly. Doubtless we always act with the best of intentions, and yet later it transpires that we did things wrong. And then we have to take responsibility for it – though this does not mean we must blame and condemn ourselves.

So one way of taking the sting out of resentment is replacing the picture of blame with that of 'capacity' – the potential each person has, given the various limitations we all carry and the many different problems we are all dealing with.

An exercise: sending good thoughts

At first this exercise may seem false or over-pious, but if you genuinely try it, the results for your emotional state can be powerful. Perhaps try it experimentally at first.

Think of someone you actively dislike, someone you feel great anger towards or someone who has done you harm. Your mind will want to run down its accustomed track listing their actions and registering the harm inside you. Instead, try to send them good thoughts. Try to cultivate vivid positive thoughts about the person and then imagine those good feelings winging their way to them.

We can send out positive thoughts to a great many people, and also to the natural world and the whole planet. When we are able to take time and do this seriously, many people feel this exercise does them a great deal of good.

Try to be open to what happens in consequence, whatever develops or arises from these loving thoughts.

This is a very difficult exercise. We are trying to generate thoughts and feelings other than those that spontaneously arise. But when we set aside blame and condemnation, even temporarily, and find positive thoughts, we develop great inner strength, and this will stand us in good stead.

Understanding our negative experiences differently

It is a great gift to have people around us who lovingly tell us, without blame or disparagement, what effect our action or behaviour had on them. It helps us become more self-aware and to recognise the consequences of our actions. How can we otherwise learn or develop?

I think it would often help if we could admit both to ourselves and to others that we did what we did in the only way we could at the time. What followed from it was unfortunate or wrong, but it was all we could do at that time.

Our own life experience determines how we see and interpret things, how we think about them. One of my teachers, Bernard C.J. Lievegoed, expressly pointed us in this direction, saying that life is determined not by what happens outwardly to us, but by our inner responses. Not *what* we experience, but how we deal with what we experience is critical.

It is hard to let go of blame and of the wrongs that have been done to us. But if we can shift from judgement, then we refuse to keep the wrong alive. Keeping it alive is damaging to everyone involved, including ourselves.

An exercise: standing in the other person's shoes

In this exercise, we try to imagine being the person we are angry with, the person who has done us harm. Or we try to imagine standing where they stand, in their position in the situation, and in their life.

What does the world look like from where they are?

We cannot ever be confident we see into another person's situation, and yet this exercise, when done with good intention, may reveal unexpected insights.

We may come to understand, perhaps, a little of the other person's feelings in a way we couldn't before.

On doing this exercise, one of my patients described realising that she and the person she was so angry with had quite particular similarities. She found tendencies in herself that were the same as those in the person who harmed her. This helped her manage her resentment.

Choosing how we respond to wrongs

It is possible to suffer terrible wrongs and yet not become stuck in rage, hate or thoughts of revenge. Inside each of us there is a source of great positivity. We do not have to react in expected or automatic ways when we are wronged. If we draw on the power of light we bear within us we can overcome our initial reaction and develop calm and equanimity.

Forming good, loving thoughts whatever the circumstances is something everyone can do, but we have to practise.

A story: a meeting in Rwanda

In Rwanda, there was a gathering of many people from different tribes and ethnicities who had fought bitterly with each other. The meeting was called with the express purpose of finding some basis for reconciliation. The mediator, Marshall Rosenberg, came to one of my seminars and spoke about the process. He said that the conversation at that gathering included people who were known to have murdered family members of others there. Marshall Rosenberg reported that some of the latter harboured thoughts of revenge, but many others were filled with a quite different impulse: their only wish was to do everything in their power to prevent such a thing ever happening again.

A story: deciding not to hate

This story comes to us through George Ritchie, an American soldier in the Second World War. At the end of the war, Ritchie was part of a division tasked with winding up a German concentration camp. An inmate of the camp was assigned to help him.

This inmate, we will call him 'the mediator', was a person who was always called on when disputes needed settling. Ritchie and the mediator worked very hard. The mediator seemed tireless. He kept thinking of this or that person in the camp who would need help of some kind.

There were many fierce and unpleasant disputes between the inmates, and the mediator would help to resolve them. One day, after yet another one of these severe arguments, Ritchie said to the mediator he could well understand the inmates' level of anger and fractiousness after everything they had been through.

The mediator did not seem to agree. He started telling Ritchie about his life.

He had been a lawyer, living and working in Warsaw when the German army invaded. He was Jewish. Before his eyes, the soldiers had put his wife and four children up against the wall and shot them. He had begged the soldiers to kill him too. But they said they needed him as an interpreter because he spoke such good German.

The mediator told Ritchie that at that moment he realised he had a choice. The soldiers had just robbed him of all that was precious to him. Now he was free to decide whether to hate them. As a lawyer he had seen what hate did to people, and so he decided to love all those he met for the rest of his life, however long it might last.[54]

Resentment and anger reduce our capacity to heal

Resentment, rage and hate constrain and consume us. If we don't try to overcome these negative emotions, the forces being consumed within us are not available for our recovery. We spend great energy on our negative frame of mind instead.

A person's inner peace resonates directly with the immune system. Immunological processes are closely related to our inner state and psyche.

The process of forgiveness

German Benedictine author Anselm Grün once wrote about forgiveness, describing it as a process.

Many say, 'You're a Christian, you have to forgive.' There's a kind of pressure in this idea: I *must* forgive. I *shouldn't* be angry.

Yet forgiveness is a process that requires time and feeling and thought.

The first step in the process is to allow yourself to feel pain.

'This hurt me. I do not judge the other, but it did hurt.' I allow myself to feel the hurt.

The second step is to allow yourself to feel anger. Anger is the power to cast out something alien from your own self. I need distance from the person who hurt me.

The third step is to perceive objectively what actually happened. If I do this then perhaps I can understand. Perhaps the other person was only passing on their own wounds, or simply touched on my own raw nerve – a place where others had hurt me before – and that's why I felt so hurt. So, I need to understand. I can only be steadfast in regard to something I understand.

The fourth step is forgiveness itself. I liberate myself from the negative energy that remains in me from the hurt. Forgiveness is a therapeutic act. I acknowledge to myself that I can be the way I am. And I stay close to myself. I free myself from the other person's power.

The fifth step is to transform the wound into a pearl, and to recognise that through the injury I gained my pearl.[55]

An exercise: letting go of anger with a loving picture

Picture a person you have been in conflict with, or a person you have been feeling angry towards.

Then try to imagine that person having a loving or joyful experience. Try to make this picture as vivid as you can. The old picture of their faults will keep interposing itself, and it will take some effort for you to maintain an image of their loving connection with life. But in this way you will practise letting go of the fixed 'shadow picture' of the other person, which may be harming both you and them.

It is especially helpful to practise this exercise before you fall asleep, and thus take the loving picture into the night with you.

Forgiving the dead

How can I forgive someone who has died? People often ask this question. I don't believe that the world of expanded awareness, the world of the spirit – the world that those who have had near-death experiences have briefly visited – is separate from us.

Perhaps we are closer to accessing this world when we sleep. The old wisdom tells us that 'sleeping on a problem' can help bring answers. Why not take your need to forgive into the night? Perhaps the following day you will receive some kind of help or answer, if you are able to attend carefully to your inner processes. It is my belief that in this other world, the dead do indeed experience us if they wish to. And so we can carry our wish to forgive or be forgiven closer to this realm as we fall asleep.

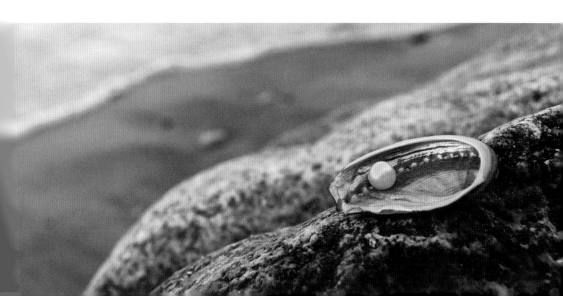

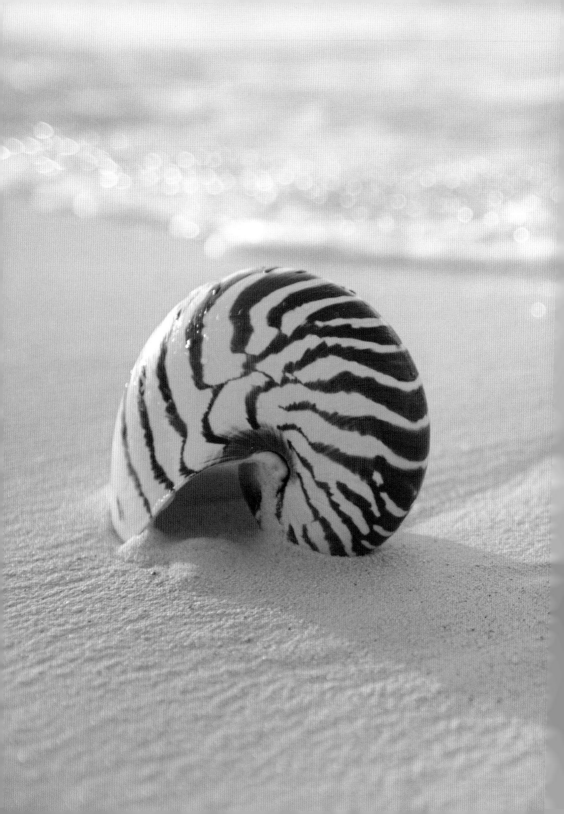

Before I entered this earthly life,
I saw a vision of how the years would be:
all the anxiety and strife,
the sorrows, suffering and misery.
I saw the vices that would grip me tight,
all the errors that would make me lame:
swift anger, resentment at my fate,
and hate and arrogance, and shame.

But I saw too the joyfulness of days
filled to the brim with lovely dreams and light,
where grievances and torment have made way
for knowledge of the grace and gifts we get
from a deep source: where love flows to the soul
still bound in earthly garb from human beings
   who now
are freed from human agonies, made whole
to serve the lofty spirits that they know.

A vision was shown me of the good and bad,
I saw the wound from which I bleed:
the full extent of all my flaws and lack,
but also the angels' helping deeds.
And as I looked there on my future life,
I heard a being ask me if I dared
to live it, for the hour had now arrived
to make this decision and descend.

And weighing up all the pain and wrong again,
I gave my certain answer, 'This is the life that I
intend to live!' And so I embarked upon
this new existence and its destiny.
And so I was born upon this earth
and do not lament when all things seem
to conspire against me, since, before my birth,
I saw them all before me and affirmed them.

Anon

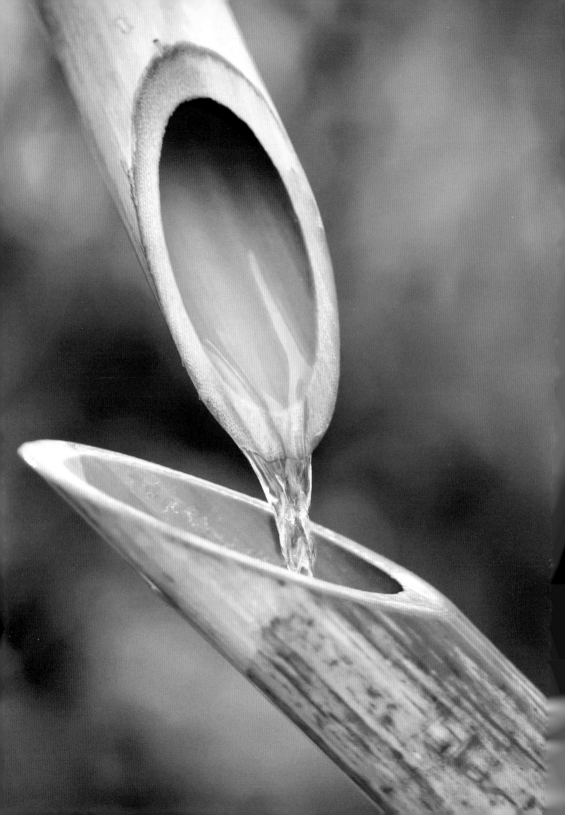

Wider Causes and Meanings

Does this illness have a meaning?

Some patients have a clear sense of the meaning of illness in their lives, amounting almost to certain knowledge. They ascribe their illness to unhappy circumstances such as long-lasting stress, worries, care, grief, negative changes in life, in their family (separation, conflict, loss), or at work. They recognise that at some point these things became too much for them.

In some, this knowledge leads to courage and trust: they find certainty that they can make the changes they need to restore equilibrium and health.

Others, who likewise see what caused their illness, find it impossible to see how change could come about. 'I can't go on. But I can't change anything either. It's hopeless.'

To these patients I say gently that even if we can't alter outer circumstances, perhaps we can change our inner stance.

Other people find no answer to the question 'Why?' They look back on their past and can see no cause. But perhaps the meaning of the illness is about the present and future, not the past. Perhaps these people need to ask not 'Why?' but 'What for?'

It may be that an illness has many consequences, and many possible meanings. It may be that some aspects of the illness are good, as well as aspects that are bad. Sometimes, indeed, illness can help us become the person we really wish to be.

Heartfelt dialogue at the time of death

I am so often deeply moved when accompanying people at the very end of their lives. Gratitude and humility rise up in me when I witness how they become able to engage in heartfelt dialogue, and express their deepest selves.

For instance, I have seen how two people were able to lovingly say what their experience of the other has been, and, without any blame or recrimination, tell how the other's behaviour affected them, what they felt, and what they would have wished for. Such a conversation, founded on this inner authenticity, which states how things were without judging them, is deeply healing.

Close to the threshold of death, a conversation of this kind enlarges love and peace in all those involved. It becomes possible to look away from the fragility of 'Brother Ass', as Francis of Assisi called the physical body, and meet inwardly, soul to soul: a loving encounter of one 'I' with another.

I have repeatedly seen how strengthening it can be, and how inner peace develops, when a person no longer defines themselves in terms of their body but as a free and living spiritual being.

Many people say that the moment they can no longer dwell easily within the body, they have an out-of-body experience, a different form of consciousness in which they have other capacities of perception and insight.

If in the midst of our life here on Earth we could entrust to one another our authentic truth and deeply felt experiences, as those close to death seem able to do, this would foster peace between people.

A peaceful death

We cannot hope to die peacefully if our lives have been full of violence, or if our minds have mostly been agitated by emotions like anger, attachment and fear. So if we wish to die well, we must learn how to live well: hoping for a peaceful death, we must cultivate peace in our mind, and in our way of life.[56]

The Dalai Lama

Causes beyond our individual lives

Many patients wonder about the root of their illness. In doing so they focus primarily on the time from diagnosis back to their birth, but often an answer is not forthcoming.

I invite you to consider the possibility that the period in which this cause originated might reach back much further. In my work with many patients I get the feeling that we bring an individual destiny with us at birth. Some patients have a clear sense of this and are convinced there is wider meaning at work in their lives, even if they cannot pinpoint a cause for their illness.

If you can find sense in the idea that there is purposefulness and wisdom in your illness and in your destiny, try also entertaining the thought that a 'cause' may lie in the distant past but could also approach from the future.

Finding wider meanings in illness

Sometimes it is very apparent how a single person's life-changing illness instigates changes and developments within them and among those around them, and opens opportunities which might otherwise never have been seen.

I frequently hear relatives and others who accompany the dying expressing their gratitude for this period because of its focus on essentials. They have gained a change in outlook and recognised the intensity of experience. These changes around a patient might point us towards a quite different form of 'causation', a cause above and beyond an individual person's experience.

From our current, limited perspective, we may not discern all the purposes at work in the great wisdom of life.

We know from watching life through the years that some events or blows of fate to do not fully reveal their meaning until many years later. Or perhaps they only do in a future life. If we recall the near-death experiences we have read about, and include such experiences in our reflections, it is possible that a whole new dimension of meaning may open up for us.

In this context I was particularly moved by something Sabine Mehne said about her near-death experience. She saw her whole life before her as a great panorama. She was able to look upon every situation in her life, with all those with whom she was connected in each situation, and feel what these people had felt and thought. This gave her insight, she said, into the meaning of each occurrence in her life. Things she had failed to understand previously were suddenly comprehensible to her because she had perceived the thoughts and feelings of others.[57]

Destinies

Have I not always eternally chosen all my destinies?[58]

Novalis

Is illness the problem, the symptom or the cure?

One of my art therapy tutors, Dr. Friedrich Lorenz, an old, very wise physician, said: 'The illness cures the cause of the illness.'

We would assuredly regard a great many illnesses differently if we could see with more inward eyes what the illness is healing.

We need to understand the widest context of any illness before we can know whether it is beneficial or not.

Take fever, for example. We all have a normal body temperature, and if it rises and we have a fever, we might worry about the change and think we have to bring our temperature down quickly by taking a tablet. And yet the cause of fever may be bacteria that have invaded the body, and our body is actively combating and vanquishing the invasion. Thus the body, the organism, perceives an unhealthy occurrence, and sends its organising forces, its healing forces, to remedy the disorder. In doing so it engenders heat – a fever – which is healing since it helps re-establish the body's original, healthy state.

What happens if we interpret fever as an illness instead of as a process of healing? The body's self-healing process is interrupted as soon as we suppress the fever. In some life-threatening situations, of course, this can be absolutely necessary. But the generalised view that we should never have a temperature is a very dubious outlook in the long term. If we suppress a beneficial fever we weaken our immune system.

How do I make peace with myself, with my situation, with my fate, with God? We make peace by finding meaning, or trusting that there is meaning, in our lives – including in our illnesses.

What it is

It is nonsense
says reason.
It is what it is,
says love.

It is disaster,
says calculation,
it is nothing but pain,
says fear,
it is hopeless
says intelligence.
It is what it is,
says love.

It is ridiculous,
says pride,
it is foolish,
says caution,
it is impossible,
says experience.
It is what it is,
says love.

Erich Fried

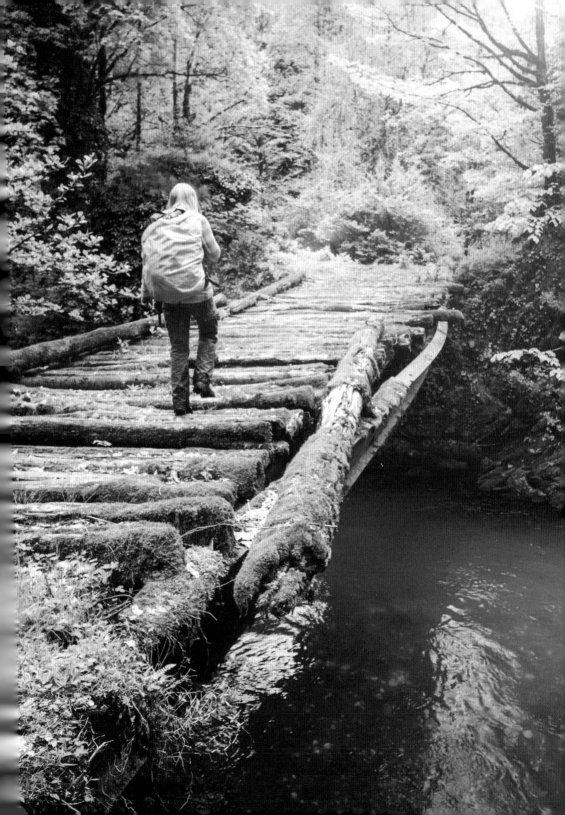

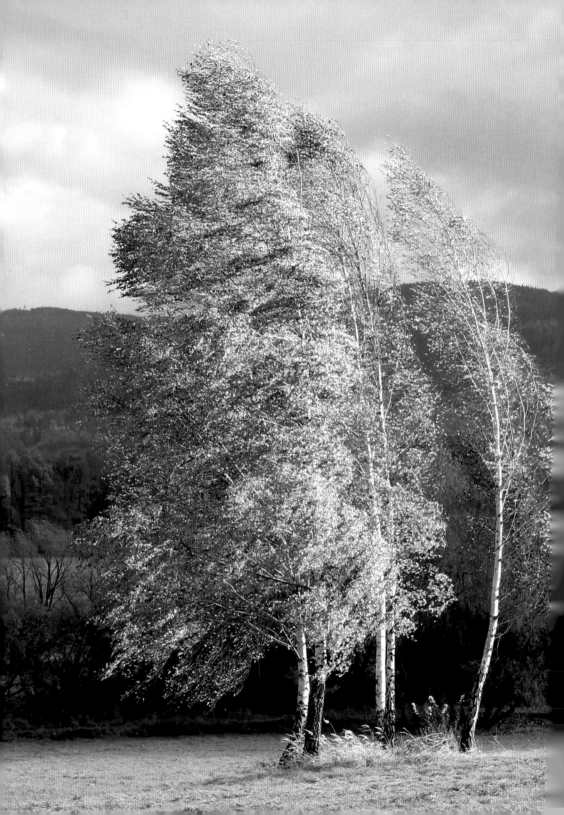

Wind, what would you be
without trees to sigh in?
Spirit, what would you be
without bodies for a dwelling?

All life wants to meet resistance.
All light wants gloom.
All weather wants tree trunk and wall
to beat against,
and practise upon.

Christian Morgenstern

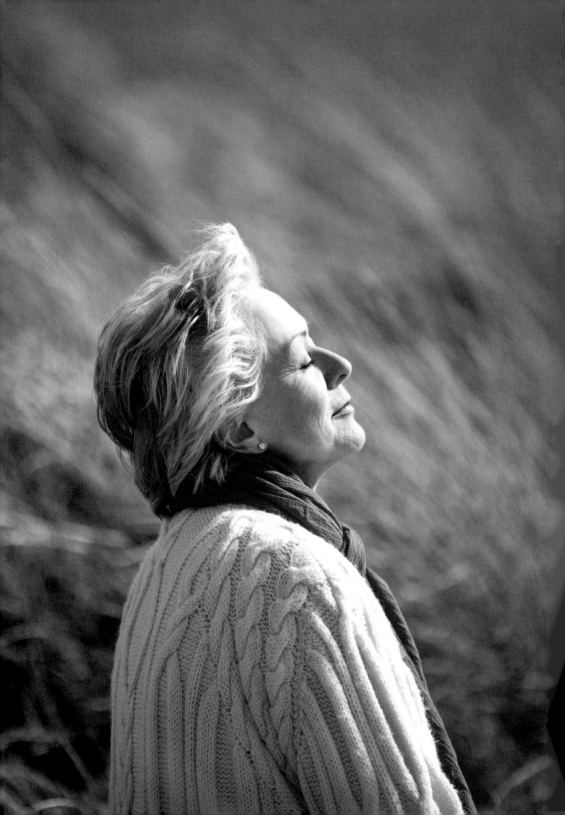

Overcoming Inner Resistance

Resisting recovery

Each time we go to the doctor, we hope that we will be met with good intuitions, ideas and suggestions, that we will benefit from supportive medicine. And yet not every patient can always and immediately answer 'Yes!' to the question of whether they *really* want to recover. This may sound very odd. Of course everyone wants to get better, you might say. And yet we also know that we often work against our own health, despite the desire for it. Our choices are often unhealthy.

Which aspect of us should we actually believe? The part of us that says it wants to be healthy, or the part that acts in ways that are anything but? Faust says, 'Two souls there are, alas, within my breast.' If the first soul is reason and mind, the other might be habit, drive, short-term enjoyment.

All of us battle with bad habits, but we can get a grip on them, or let go of them altogether, and we are often aided in this by pain or illness. We have the capacity to learn – slowly, and with practice – to act out of insight and knowledge.

Why 'just functioning' can be bad for us

Our body, as we know, is a kind of instrument for shaping our lives, and is imbued with a wisdom beyond our understanding. Its power to heal is incalculable: it heals itself every day like an ongoing miracle.

But the body, like the soul and spirit, needs our attention and care to be healthy. In the era we inhabit, we are increasingly attentive to many things we once would not have known about. Modern media makes us aware of everything happening in the world, but it also offers us such a wealth of possibilities, so many calls on our attention, that it is no longer so easy to focus on essentials. In the modern world it is all too easy to lose ourselves and be distracted.

Many patients say they have lost sight of who they are, of their own needs, in their busy lives caring for many other people and living out multiple roles. Of course, we have all kinds of relationships with people, involving tasks and duties. We are not just here for ourselves. But we do need to cultivate a dialogue with ourselves, since, if we lose touch with who we are, this easily becomes unhealthy. If we 'just function' this means doing things without real joy, enthusiasm and meaning, it means that we suppress ourselves, cannot 'breathe' properly, and we cease to feel we are really ourselves.

If we merely function, or are constantly distracted with extraneous things, it is likely that we are no longer open to a sudden flash of inspiration. Our 'antennae' are not receiving, we are no longer open for intuitions about the next step, the way forward in life. When we merely function, it is likely that moments of real happiness will become ever more rare.

When we merely function, we are like a machine that can't feel. And if we can no longer feel who we are, how can we take full responsibility for ourselves? It seems to me that we have, in this case, relinquished ourselves to some degree, and are no longer at home in ourselves. If you leave a house uninhabited for long enough, it starts to collapse.

Questions: enthusiasm, inspiration and joy

❀ What gives you the strength to act?

❀ What is it that lovingly connects you with life, enthuses and fulfils you?

❀ You have great creative potential within. Can you think of a way to get in touch with it?

I suggest trying something new, something that appeals to you that you haven't done before. Inspiring new experiences transform habitual modes of thought in our brain. They can become the 'magic key' to unlocking the change we desire.[59]

❀ When are you entirely at home in yourself?

❀ When are you connected to the world in love and gratitude?

❀ What inspires and enthuses you? What really speaks to you?

❀ When was the last time you felt childlike vitality, the joy in existence that is so innate in children?

If we can keep recreating loving, joyful connection with life, the strength we discover at such moments will grow.

Time for building

We all build our own house, metaphorically speaking. Imagine you are a builder who has been told there will be a flood in the next few days. You would likely expend all your strength and energy on defending the house you've built so far. Probably you would stop adding to the rooms for living and construct a protective wall.

As soon as our external activities assume proportions that no longer leave sufficient energy for building and sustaining our own body, our body will stagnate and suffer. We need to recognise what is happening and re-establish equilibrium.

Perceiving our own needs

At the Eschelbronn Clinic where I ran seminars, we would talk about the difference between life at Eschelbronn and daily life.

With nods of agreement from others, one woman said, 'Here at Eschelbronn, I perceive my own needs, and my needs are perceived.'

If we want to regain our health we need daily life to become much more like life at Eschelbronn. If we want to nurture our healing forces we have to work to be present and 'at home' in ourselves.

What hinders our care for ourselves?

Many patients say that daily life prevents them from fulfilling their own needs. Some say they know exactly what they need, but it's impossible to arrange for it among other pressures, at home or at work.

Others talk of a voice inside that pushes them. One patient spoke of a little devil who drives her. It sits on her shoulder and says all the time: 'Come on, get on with it, keep functioning!'

Most often, though, we founder because we overtax ourselves, trying to do too much in too short a time.

There are also our expectations of life, of ourselves. Do we sometimes push too hard for life to be other than it is? Do we sometimes imagine our path in life should be broad and straight? So often reality is different. The Spanish poet Antonio Machado wrote: '*Caminante, no hay camino, se hace camino al andar...*' Traveller, there is no path but the one you make by walking...[60]

Choosing openness over security

Our dogmatic ideas are a great obstacle to overcoming inner resistance and learning to live more authentically and autonomously.

We all have thoughts and ideas that have become engrained. They can give us security but they can also prevent us from being open to life's reality and from recognising our own needs.

Medical dogma

Perhaps surprisingly, we also meet dogmatic ideas in scientific research circles. There are many studies of psycho-oncology, for example, and they point in both negative and positive directions. Despite the evidence being so finely balanced, I am struck by the general medical conclusion that psycho-oncology must therefore have no benefits. Is this a truly scientific spirit and a genuine openness to new ideas? It seems that scientific research is not free from preconceptions.

Dr Gunver Kienle, of the Institute for Applied Epistemology and Medical methodology describes the goal of a 'patient-centred medicine':

> The Institute of Medicine in the USA regards patient-centred medicine (which we can also call 'subject-oriented medicine') as one of the most important aims for twenty-first-century medical research and practice. Hitherto we have had an 'it medicine', positioning the patient as object rather than subject. Complementary medical research shows that patient-centred medicine is not a luxury but is more economical, even, than 'it

medicine'... But people ignore these studies. I have rarely come across critics who had any real sense of the available research and study findings. Most simply assert there is nothing to demonstrate its value. But globally there are around 2,000 studies on complementary medicine, with an incredible wealth of research and meta-analysis. It's simply being ignored.[61]

A story: refusing new ideas

The mid-eighteenth century offers a sad and salutary example of the inability of medical practice to embrace new ideas.

A great many women used to die of fever after giving birth. Then a young physician, Dr Ignaz Philipp Semmelweis, had a brainwave: he noticed that there were many more deaths on wards attended by doctors who were also attending patients with diseases than on wards attended by midwives who dealt exclusively with women giving birth. He suggested that doctors should always wash their hands when they attended births, especially if they went straight there from conducting post mortems. He was the first, therefore, to conceive of the idea of disinfection.

But there was no understanding of germs or bacteria to explain his ideas and most doctors dismissed them. Many more years were to pass before the need for hygiene was introduced in medical practice. Once it was adopted widely, huge numbers of lives were saved.

Semmelweis died tragically in a lunatic asylum at the age of 47.

An exercise: looking back mindfully

In the evening, before you fall asleep, look back on the past day in reverse, from the evening back to the morning.[62]

This exercise asks for presence of mind: it strengthens mindfulness, helping you to be present in the moment. In looking back on the day you can call to mind the situations that you especially valued, as well as those that didn't go so well. Gaining some distance from what has happened, you can reflect on ways to do better next time, and when a similar situation recurs, you may be able to deal with it better, and with greater awareness.

Thinking backwards disconnects us from our usual analyses and assumptions, from our accepted ideas of cause and effect. It allows us to see what is, without leaping to judgment, and so gives us time to step back and reflect. This is an opportunity to get in touch with yourself and your feelings.

When you know what you feel, you may discover that your life has grown unbalanced in some way. Then you can consider what would be needed to re-establish balance.

Obstacles in the medical system

Besides our personal preconceptions, another obstacle impeding our recovery can be the focus of the medical world on 'repair' and the suppression of symptoms. When we go along with this in our own thinking, we internalise a systemic obstacle and it can become another fixed idea that blocks our way.

In acute wards we have created conditions where the prime focus is on alleviating and eradicating the most apparent symptoms as quickly as possible. There is no longer time in the health system for understanding underlying causes and working in longer-term and more sustainable ways. While this focus on acute symptoms has saved the lives of many people, it often fails to ask what is needed to initiate deeper, fundamental processes of healing.

Interest in what can produce a real and lasting cure also gets drowned out by a functionalism in which each medical professional has their specific, allotted task. As doctors specialise in narrower fields, they may lose sight of the factors that bring healing to the whole organism.

'Symptom management' is vital, but it offers no guarantee that the patient's organic processes will be reconfigured in a healthier way. In many cases we see that the removal of symptoms does not automatically signify a cure. I have known patients to receive a transplant only to find that their disease forms again in the new organ just as it did in the old one. A whole developmental process underlies the appearance of a symptom, and simply removing the symptom is often not enough.

Sometimes it seems that the principle of studying what works, so widely accepted elsewhere, does not figure sufficiently in medicine. Have we perhaps created a quite new, narrow definition of success in this system? Have we developed a language that allows us to conceal from ourselves the difference between removal of symptoms and a successful cure?

It seems to me that investigating why some patients recover despite poor medical prognoses would be a very worthy field of study. It is one that is currently much neglected. People who defy all prognoses are often simply dismissed as 'lucky'. Isn't it rather strange that we speak of 'spontaneous remission', without reflecting more thoroughly on what those patients have been doing, their inner and outer activity?

If we exclude from consideration the active contribution of patients to their own recovery, we do not reflect the full reality. This stance overlooks patient competency and limits healing to medical intervention alone. This is, surely, a narrow and limiting outlook.

Shall we acknowledge that all the healthy changes a patient makes can

234

have a significant effect on remission of their disease? Are we willing to acknowledge that those who recover despite adverse prognoses may owe this to some degree to their will for life and deep faith in recovery?

A story: Lillian and the incurious doctor

I have a personal example of a particular lack of medical curiosity.

My first grandchild, Lillian, was born with stage III osteogenesis imperfecta, or brittle bone disease. Her bones are therefore very fragile. She lives in Sacramento, California, and at the age of three underwent surgical implants of telescopic nails in her upper thigh bones. The very experienced surgeon said to my daughter, 'In the past, when operating on all children with the same severity of this condition as your daughter, I have always been able to scratch the bone with a scalpel, and it was porous. But in your daughter's case I needed a drill and I had to use pressure. I don't know what you've been doing, but it has helped!'

Yet very strangely, he didn't go on to ask her *what* she had been doing! It was as if he had no interest in enquiring further. Why didn't he ask? I wish he had! Perhaps he was so focused on his specialism that he had lost sight of an interest in how health can be strengthened.

A patient's agency in recovery

Medical intervention and support is often life-saving and lengthens survival time, but to see it as the only means of a cure would, in my view, be as risky as thinking the mind alone can heal. Together, both medical science and the power of the mind and spirit can open up all sorts of possibilities.

The patient, the one who is ill, should be the chief protagonist in recovery, and the words we use should accentuate this. Yet we often use terms that disempower patients, or make them into a number for ease of codification. There should be no doubt that the patient is central, and all administration of their care must serve healing. If this is not the case, we find ourselves in a pathological situation in which an administrative spirit governs our 'places of healing'. Then the 'health system' is, in fact, ailing.

An exercise: how much recovery is due to the patient?

Consider the question: what percentage of any recovery do you feel is due to the ill person themselves, and how much would you attribute to medicine?

It is very interesting to see how differently people answer this question.

Most patients give themselves a share in recovery of between 30 and 90 per cent.

No one has yet said to me that medicine is entirely responsible for curing a person. It seems we all recognise that we have some part to play in our healing.

I found the answer a pharmacologist gave me especially interesting. She said, 'If you ask me the question as a pharmacologist, I'd say the patient themselves plays a 20 per cent part in their cure. But now I myself have had cancer for two years, it has all turned upside down. Now I'd say 80 per cent of recovery is due to the patient and only 20 per cent to medicine!'

Belief in our powers of recovery

Recovery at the physiological and biochemical level does need medical support, but it can only occur if the body, and the body's own healing and reorganising powers, take on their own work and activity again. This is the mechanism for lasting recovery.

It sometimes seems to me that our degree of openness to reality is a sure measure of whether we have embarked on a path towards health. We can see illness as a time of learning. We face the challenge of developing thinking that accords with reality. This includes a belief in our power of recovery.

Many people are only alive because of medical intervention, but keeping a person alive is not the same as helping them to stay healthy.

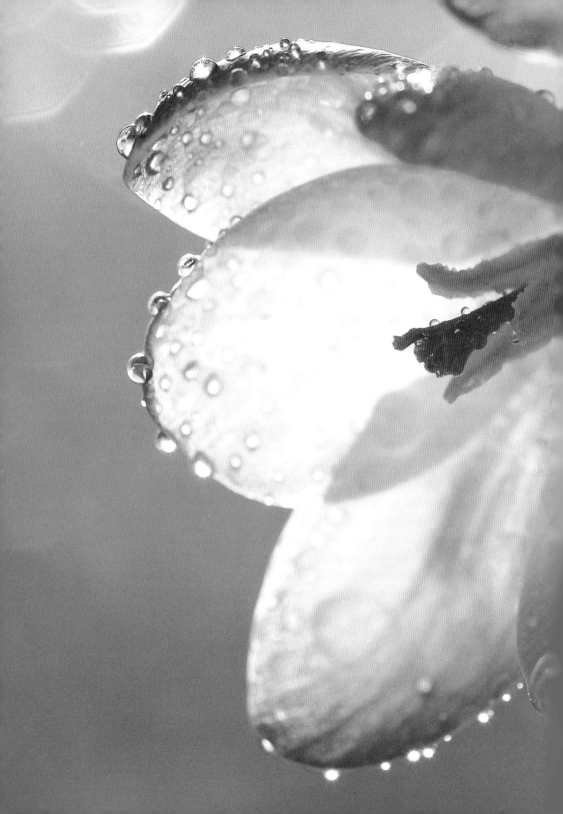

Certainty

Whence, in the fearful depths of night
comes such sweet comfort to me,
from what higher power of heart
streams such tranquillity?

It seems as if a feathery wing
brushed down in heavenly breeze,
as if my heart in joyous spring
heard childhood's melodies.

It seems as if I floated free
through blessed meadows bright,
as if dawned vast against the sky,
an unknown image on my sight.

As yet I'm deaf to this dark call,
blind yet to such bright light,
but he who made me deaf and blind, I feel
will stay by me this night.

Paul Jaeger

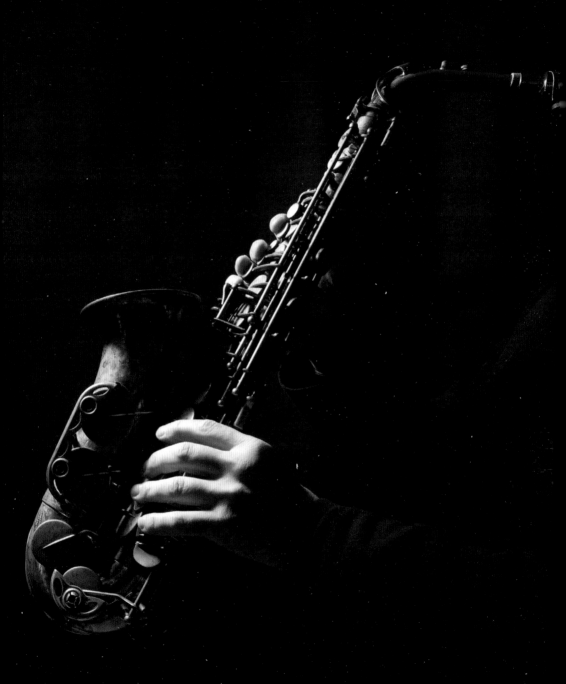

The Person
I Really Am

Outer and inner experiences

Both outer and inner experiences have a reality to which we can attend. Some people lead a more outward-oriented life; others – monks are a particular instance – prioritise a more meditative path focused on inner contemplation. We all live between these two planes of reality and must keep finding the right balance between them.

But often the external world elicits our sharpest attention. As children we learn very early what we have to do to gain the love, acknowledgement and esteem we all long for, and which is so important for our growth and development. Over time this quest or longing for external acknowledgement may sometimes mean that we lose sight of our own path.

The danger of losing oneself

We can lose ourselves in any activity or distraction or relationship. The existential question, then, is whether we are simply completely absorbed in it, or whether we have become enslaved by it.

Many people looking back to the time before their illness recognise that they were no longer fully themselves, they were 'just functioning'.

In other words, we can live our lives without being fully present, without completely owning them.

Lawrence LeShan, a pioneer of psycho-oncology, has spoken of a person losing the 'melody of their life'.[63] His work primarily focused on giving people the help and support they needed to learn to hear this melody again, and act upon it.

With his help, 50 per cent of patients who had been deemed incurable recovered. From this we can grasp that health is not purely a biochemical issue. We can see that the release and nurturing of healing forces in us can be intimately connected with our capacity to be ourselves.

Being who we really are

Surely the deepest longing in our hearts is to be the person we really are. Or, to put it differently, to become the person we can be. And how deeply gratifying if, at the end of our lives, we can look back and say 'I was the person I was meant to be.'[64]

Dr Carl Simonton said:

> One of the chief causes of illness is our attempts to be other than we are. And one of the most important health-giving steps is to turn towards who we really are.

Nothing is in vain

On the difficult quest to be true to ourselves, here is a reflection to consider. Over time, ideas like this may assist in turning uncertainty and anxiety into knowledge and trust:

* Whatever happens to me, everything I encounter on my journey through life is deeply and closely related to my true being.
* Nothing that happens is in vain.
* Everything has a deeper meaning.
* Even the most difficult situations are there to let my true being shine through.

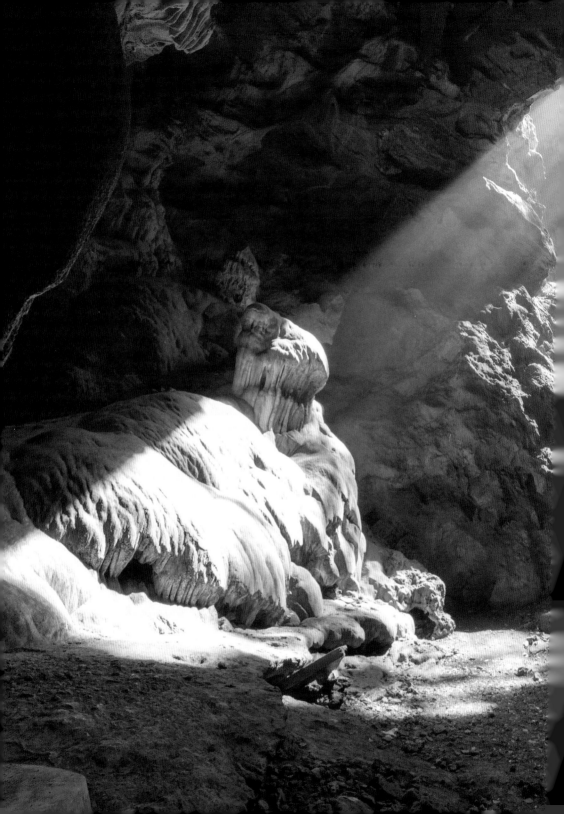

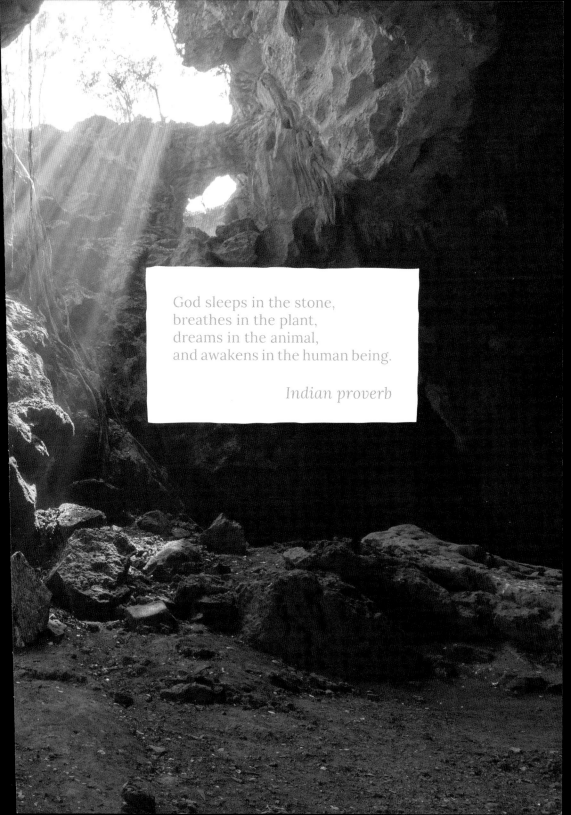

God sleeps in the stone,
breathes in the plant,
dreams in the animal,
and awakens in the human being.

Indian proverb

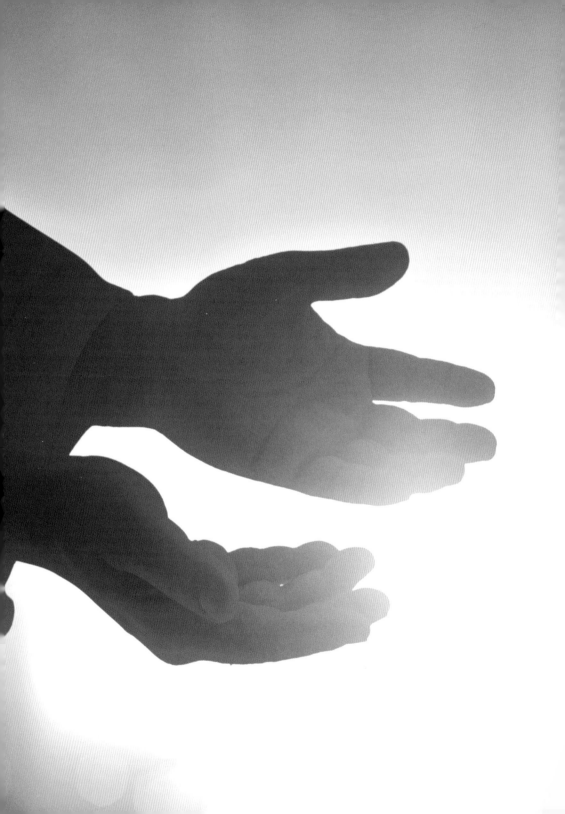

The Threefold Dialogue

Let us return now to the heart of the path of recovery, to the threefold dialogue we discussed in the very first chapter.

The moment we are faced with a serious illness, fear takes hold in many patients and their relatives. That is understandable, but we need to get beyond fear.

What distinguishes people who have overcome their fear or who no longer let it rule their lives from those who succumb to it? The inner sense of trust.

The threefold dialogue can help us transform fear. Looking back on certain situations in life, many wish they had had more 'presence of mind'. Fortunately we have the potential to direct our mind toward particular themes and issues. Goethe says, 'The animal is taught by its organs; the human being instructs and masters theirs.'[65] We can overcome fear by conducting an open dialogue with ourselves, with the other, and with the divine.

Dialogue with ourselves

Before they fell ill, the daily life of patients will often have been beset by tasks and duties, sometimes to such a degree that they may say sadly, looking back, that they lost sight of themselves. Only when they come to hospital do some people find, again, the space for a deeper encounter with themselves. And this, as we have seen, is extremely important for the healing process.

What do we nourish in ourselves and how do we do this? I myself decide what I'm interested in, what I attend to. With every decision I make I am being creatively active. My life will be determined by the degree to which I can nurture and develop my innate creative powers.

Reflection from Reinhold: not I but Christ in me

Earlier in this book I told the story of my friend Reinhold, who was told he had five months to live, but lived five years more. A priest who visited him a few weeks before his death said after the visit, 'I have never seen someone who was so well!'

The following words are from Reinhold's journal, and were written a few months before he died:

> How often we are deceived by our own ideas. We imagine things to be a particular way and pile more and more erroneous ideas on this original illusion. This is how fear arises, for instance.
>
> Fear makes you susceptible to negative powers.
>
> At such moments one has to grow beyond oneself, sunder oneself from every situation so as to find an objective, cosmic-human perspective again.
>
> You can do this by filling yourself with the thought, 'Not I but Christ in me.'
>
> Then you overcome the momentary situation: you address your own higher I. You stand freely again in life.
>
> The will that was paralysed can incarnate again. You can mobilise, and indeed discover, the forces that are available to you. ...

Noticing how we can grow alien from life, we must continually seek the centre again. And this quest is an activity that strengthens the I, consolidates it, and at the same time makes us more open. Point and periphery interpenetrate, and rhythm can arise. Rhythm is life – life shaped and configured. It is beauty in the truest sense.

This is only possible through the power of love. ... Selfless love seeks its task precisely where it is hard. ...

And selfless love fills this with the pure joy of existence, continual inner renewal, a fount of life, for the power of God works within it. And the power of God lives in us through Christ. ...

Reinhold died 'healthy' at the age of 33. In his last five years he was able to reflect and grow in ways which deeply moved all his friends. He developed a living power within, which transformed his surroundings.

He was in dialogue with the inmost core of his being.

Warmed by our own creative powers

A great many patients arrive at my art therapy studio looking disorientated and uncertain. But then something very remarkable happens. Through experiences with art therapy they discover that they are not *only* ill, but also healthy. They are healthy in other respects even while they are ill. They rediscover their creative powers. Despite their physical frailty, many leave at the end of the session with healthy red cheeks and a sense of enthusiasm. It seems to me at such moments that the person has been warmed through by their own creative power and is at home again in themselves.

Trusting ourselves

If we succeed in entering into dialogue with our deeper selves, we come to trust ourselves again. We see that we ourselves can initiate something, and that this strengthens us.

Through my respectful and loving conversation with myself, the certainty grows: 'I will take care of myself.'

Dialogue with the other

In shared experience and insight into the destiny of other patients, we come to see that we are not alone. This is a kind of 'destiny community'. While some have only just received their diagnosis, others have been facing the challenge of illness for many years and may still be finding it hard to come to terms with. In mutual perception of each other we can see the many different ways there are of coping with an illness, as well as the many kinds of support and help available.

The potential for help and healing far exceeds the scope of what is available in a clinic. Many find they can let go of the sense they have to do everything on their own, and open themselves to support from others – friends and practitioners. Then trust can grow: trust in our fellow human beings, and knowledge that even when we ourselves have reached breaking point we can still find support and succour.

People who you trust

Try to find people you trust. This is another way to enhance your own self-healing powers.

And what about your personal relationships? Do some of them demand more strength than they provide? Are some relationships fraught with underlying resentment and irritation that needs to be dealt with before you can return to open dialogue?

Dialogue with the spiritual world

Many patients feel they must make every decision and cope with everything on their own. They may feel they have no strength left to manage. Many say they have lost all belief in God and seem to be bereft of spiritual connection. They feel that if there are protective powers in the world, those powers have abandoned them.

Others tell me that in their distress they have begun to pray again. They find in themselves a certainty that they are always sustained and never abandoned. One patient put it like this: 'I cannot fall any further than into the hand of God.'

There are difficult situations in life in which we see no way forward but then suddenly feel help coming unexpectedly and surprisingly. If we can feel this we can gain trust in the benevolent guidance of a world of spirit.

The threefold dialogue

Trust in ourselves, in our fellow human beings and in the heavens soothes our anxiety. It opens the door to our own creativity, to development, change and healing. Engaging in these three forms of dialogue, we find our way to the deeper meaning of our lives.

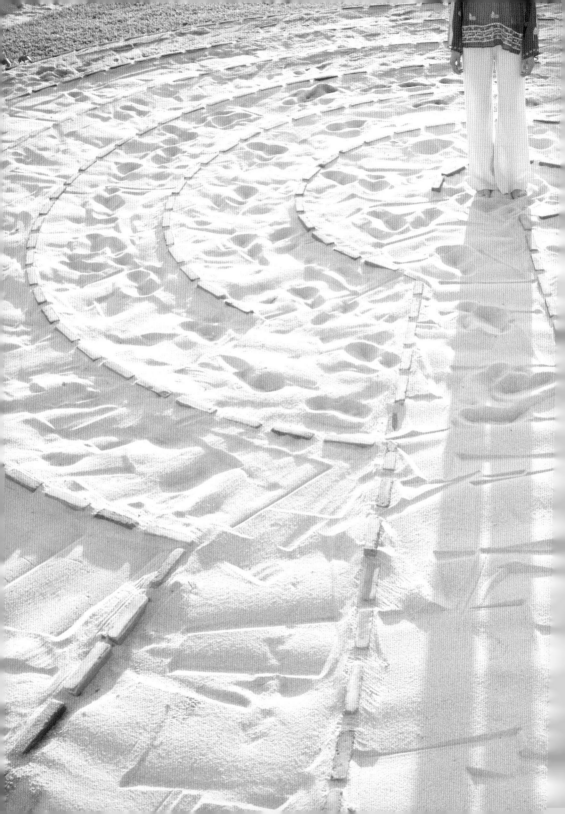

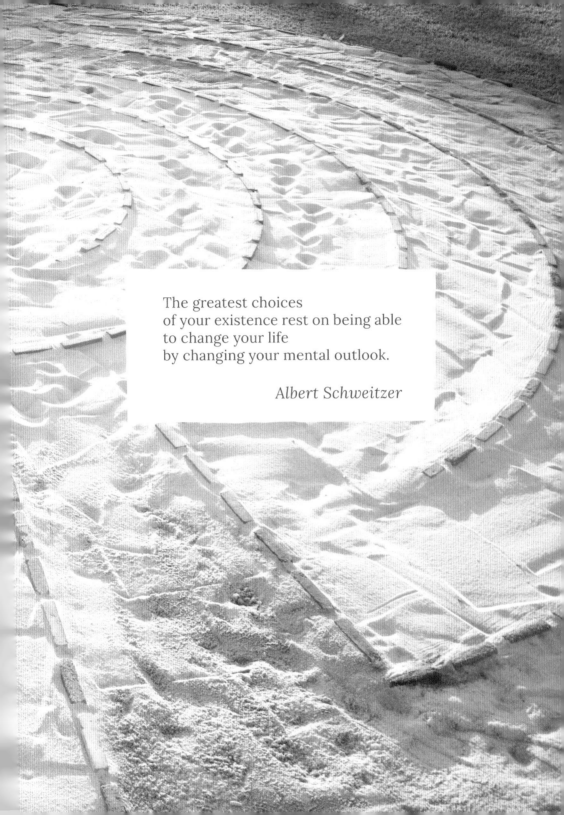

The greatest choices
of your existence rest on being able
to change your life
by changing your mental outlook.

Albert Schweitzer

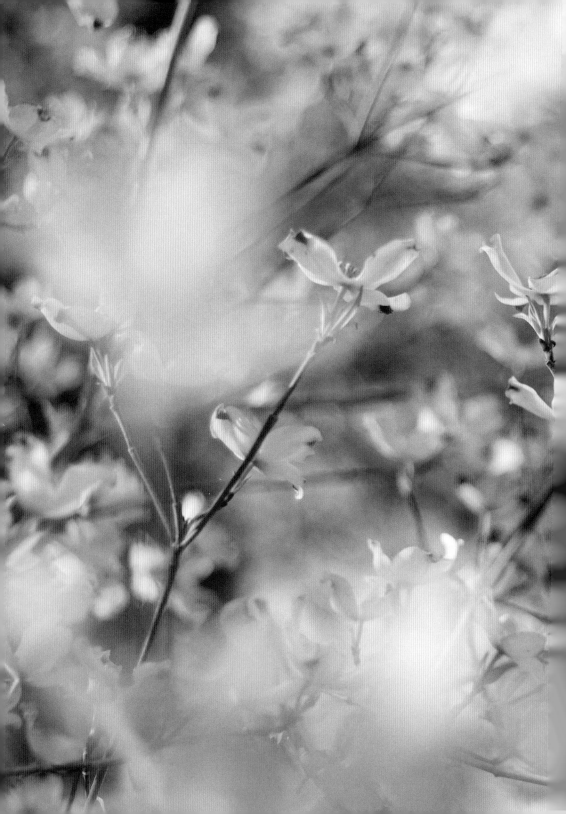

The Healing Path

What are the most important steps we have covered?

Acknowledge that healing can happen

The Swede Thomas Lindahl, who won the Nobel Prize for Chemistry, calculated that in every one of the nearly 100 billion cells in our body, defective parts of the DNA are repaired 200 times each day.[66] Here's a sum for you: if you multiply 100 billion cells by 200 defects per cell per day, and then divide this by the 86,400 seconds of every day, you can see how many curative processes occur in you every second. The numbers are almost inconceivable.

An unimaginable self-healing potential exists in us.

Recognise healing is more than biochemical

It is wilfully reductionist to limit our sense of bodily repair to machine-like technical processes over which we have no influence.

Decide to live

Deciding to live means clarifying the following questions:

- ❋ Do I really want to live?
- ❋ Why do I want to be here on the earth?
- ❋ Which people do I feel especially happy with?
- ❋ What do I want to nurture and develop?
- ❋ How can I serve life?
- ❋ What gives me joy, meaning, enthusiasm and fulfilment?

Regain your picture of the future

When we lose our vision of the future, we lose our will to live.

I ask people who attend my health seminar why they want to live, and here are some of their answers:

- ❋ Because my wife needs me
- ❋ Because I want to laugh with my kids
- ❋ Because I want to see my grandchildren grow up
- ❋ Because I enjoy the company of other people so much
- ❋ Because I still have so many plans
- ❋ Because I want to travel and get to know the world better
- ❋ Because I want to leave more of myself behind when I go
- ❋ Because I love my life

A vision of the future can help us survive terrible times – it gives strength.

Integrate what you've learned into daily life

Once we recognise what we need, we must take small, committed, practical steps to change our habits and our everyday lives. To do this we have to perceive our own resistance, then decide how to overcome it. We have to maintain faith in our intentions. If we make a firm resolve, and actually embark on our path, then the 'good spirits' will support and accompany us.

Hope for the best, yet prepare for the worst: acknowledge death within life

Of course, not everything lies within our power. Only when we integrate death into life, and acknowledge each as intrinsic to the other, can we fully embrace our living.

Re-evaluating our thoughts about death and dying can give us strength and resolve for our path in life.

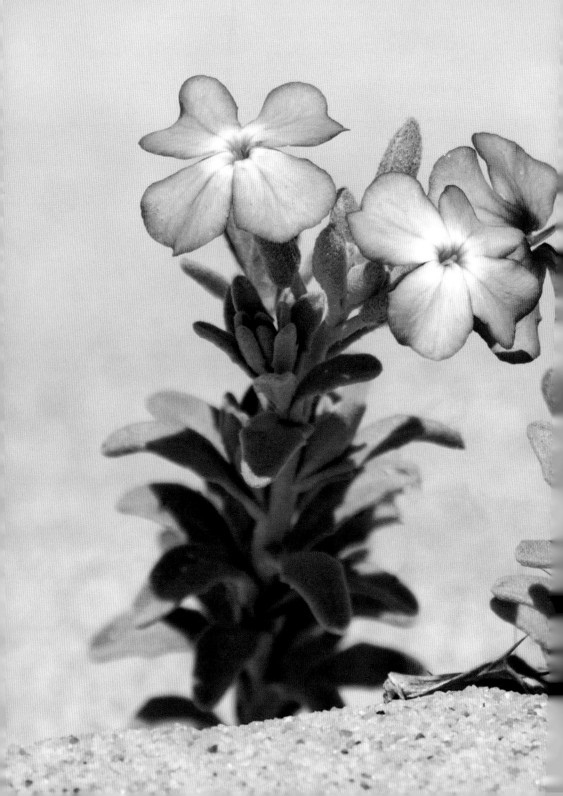

Let us take our will properly in hand and
let us seek awakening from within every
morning and every evening.

Rudolf Steiner

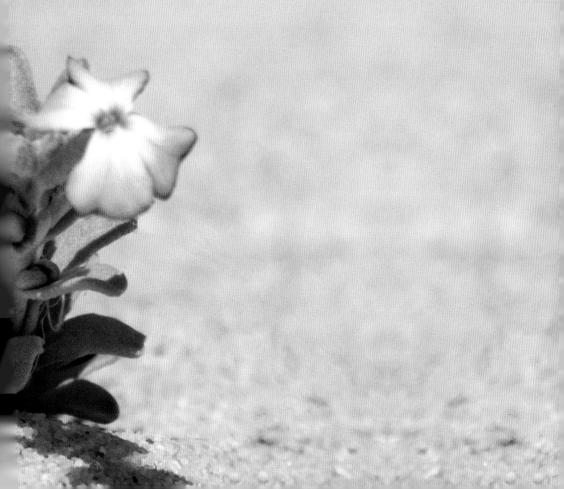

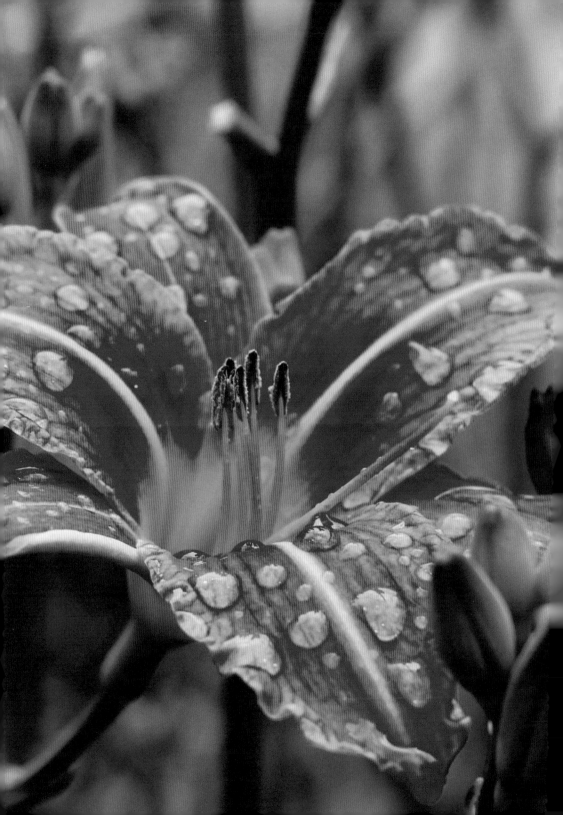

Courage for Life, Trust in Growing

To end, I want to consider three groups of people who have developed a foundation for health.

People who have had a near-death experience

The first group is people who have had a near-death experience. Such people discover that their being and consciousness does not die. They learn that death does not deprive them of life but transforms it. Their experience leads them to recognise what is truly important to them.

People diagnosed with severe illness

The second group of people have lived with a diagnosis of severe illness. Such people can discover meaning even in the most arduous circumstances. They find that illness changes them. Many say that illness has made them much more grateful toward life – grateful for themselves, their fellow human beings, nature and the world.

People who have recovered their health

The third group is people I have met in my art therapy sessions who have succeeded in recovering their health. There is a distinctive quality in these people's creative, artistic processes. They appear very open, interested and inquisitive. They have the ability to see what is actually there rather than what they imagine to be there. They have courage and trust.

Destiny is always on our side

We have all met situations which we did not want or ask for, and which have brought us a great deal of suffering. How are we supposed to regard such situations as imbued with love or wisdom? It is asking a lot – it is a lot of work – for us to acknowledge a wise, caring and loving power behind difficult events in our life. But openness to reality can help us. I have met people who succeeded in doing this. They have found an unshakeable belief that 'Destiny is never against us but always for us.'

This phrase, said to originate with Rudolf Steiner, was told me by a therapist in a clinic in Switzerland in 1982, when I was a young trainee. The thought has stayed with me ever since.

A request to oncologists

I would like to ask three things of colleagues in the health service who work in CT scan departments. The technology now available ought to mean this is possible.

1. Please give patients a graph that shows what proportion of cells in their body are healthy, and what proportion are malignant or tumour cells.

2. Please point out to patients how often these places in their body have re-organised themselves in the past and re-established health.

3. Please remind patients that they themselves, as thinking, feeling and acting human beings, have an effect on the health of their body, soul and spirit.

Illness is not a technical challenge

Medical ethicist Professor Giovanni Maio tells us:

> With all its equipment and apparatus, its access to technology, medicine offers a suggestive sense of possibility and control. This atmosphere of control through technology is attractive to patients, and almost without noticing they pass from one technical procedure to the next, unable themselves to avoid its escalation. In my view, physicians should be willing to dispense with purely technical procedures at an early enough stage, instead encouraging patients to regard illness as a task not only requiring technical solutions but as an inward challenge for them. The allure of technological feasibility prevents people from reflecting on their own powers and resources and overcoming the illness from within by incorporating it as integral to their own lives.[67]

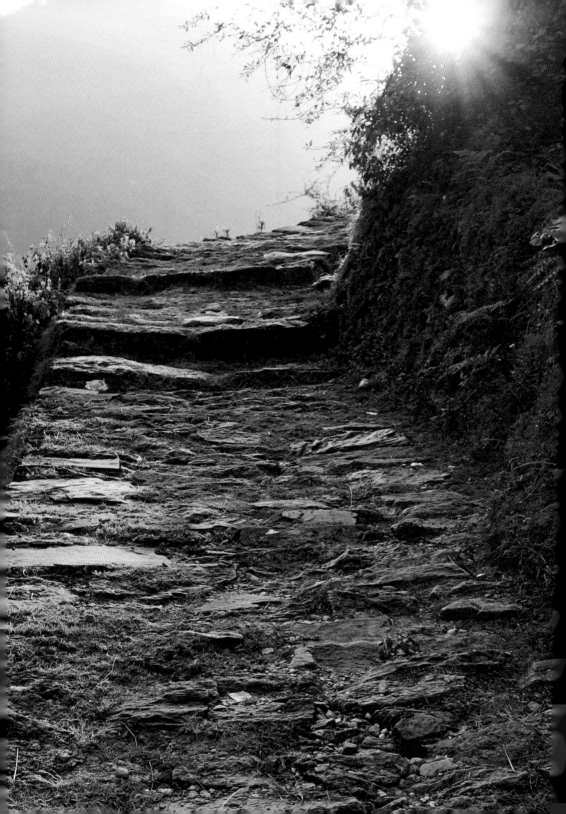

Afterword: the Cost of Medical Treatment

In cancer therapy, more and more immune system medicines are being developed, at vast expense.

The European medicines agency is releasing new active constituents onto the market nearly every month: immune therapies and medicines that promise a 'targeted' action against cancer cell mutations. The new treatments cost on average ten to forty times more than the chemotherapy they are replacing. Berlin cancer specialist Professor Wolf-Dieter Ludwig says:

> Two things are certain. In the next few years, oncology will be the field that sees most new medicines coming onto the market. And in five years time, if current trends continue, oncology medicines will represent the pharmaceutical industry's biggest sales by far – an estimated 120–40 billion US dollars globally.

Yet the outcome of such treatments is usually not a cure but an extension of survival periods by mere weeks or months. Tarceva, for example, extends survival in pancreatic cancer patients by two weeks and costs 2,353 euros per month.

If these medicines were made available to all cancer patients, some experts in the health service believe that 'our children will no longer be able to receive the healthcare we have become accustomed to'.[68] Health insurers or national health systems such as the NHS will be completely overtaxed by such developments. With this in prospect, it seems to me vital that we bring back a human scale to procedures of industrialised medicine.

Professor Christian Schubert tells us:

> The biomedical paradigm is both a blessing and a curse. Technical progress in medicine is bringing us numerous new procedures for acute problems, for instance in intensive care, transplants and reproductive medicine, and in the past has led to many other achievements such as dialysis, artificial feeding, reanimation and antibiotics treatment. Physicians and scientists can rightly be proud of all this, and patients are likewise right to feel they are in good hands. Such progress has been possible in part because science has regarded the human being as a machine, uncoupled from his social milieu – as an inert and non-subjective entity.
>
> But woe betide us if this biomedical paradigm, so successful in acute medicine, is applied to the field of chronic conditions. Its sensational successes then become a disaster. Chronic diseases such as auto-immune conditions, cancer, pain syndromes, depression and many more arise and continue in a person's relational world, and can therefore only be diagnosed and treated appropriately in that context. Psychoneuroimmunology and psychotherapy are therefore central aspects of a long-needed change of paradigm in a medicine that has for too long regarded the human being as a machine, and the clinic as a repair workshop, with direct connections to industry.[69]

This present book could not have been written without the human experience of patients in the tension between these two aspects of modern medicine, both its blessings and its curse: those who have come to see that they can shape their own individual path toward healing.

Acknowledgements

Thanks to my parents and dear brother Benno for their loving support and affirmation of me. Thanks to Regine, Annette, Rosselke, Anne, Fritz, Therese, Reiner, Hans, Renate, Bettina, Reiner, Eckard, Renee, Carl, Michael, Matthias, Christian, Markus, Ingrid Maria, Angelika, Monika, Gerald, Evelyne, Sebastian, Pamela and all the friends and teachers who stood by me on my journey, who opened doors and offered me new perspectives and experiences. Thanks to all my colleagues at the clinic who supported and encouraged me: together we discovered, learned, failed, grew, wept, laughed and prayed, all of us trying to create an environment in which people can pursue a wholesome and healing path of development. Thanks to my literary agent Volker, this book's midwife, for his far-sightedness and commitment, and to my editor for the German edition, Christine, for her enthusiasm, loving care and clarity. Likewise to Manfred Christ for his empathy in designing the German book and the cover. Thanks to my wife Susana who has supported me with tremendous positivity, joy, interest and enthusiasm, and who continually inspires me anew.

My special thanks go to all the wonderful people, the patients, whom I have been privileged to get to know and to accompany. They have taught me most. Thanks for their unconditional openness, their willingness to share what lives deep within them, their fear, rage, joy, trust, doubt, grief, hope and gratitude. Thanks for all their courage, confidence and insight, the inner certainty that they could find and follow the path that was right for them, without any ultimate assurance or guarantee. For many the greater goal is not only healing but to become, in the fullest sense, the person they wish to be. Thanks to those I accompanied who, in wrestling with all aspects of their being, at last passed over safe and whole to the other side of life with a sense of reconciliation. All these experiences fill me with humility, wonder and thankfulness for the great gift of life that we share with one another.

And then I would also like to offer thanks for the free and protected space that I have been privileged to enjoy for several decades: the scope to think and explore without preconceived or dogmatic notions imposed by ideologies or institutions – a space for perceiving, feeling and discovering, where I could pursue and develop my path in art therapy and psycho-oncology.

Thanks to all of you. You have all written this book with me.

Josef Ulrich, Eschelbronn, December 2015

Notes and References

1. Viktor E. Frankl, *Man's Search for Meaning,* Rider 2004
2. See Faith Karimi, Saeed Ahmed, 'Nelson Mandela: 10 surprising facts you probably didn't know', CNN, 6 December 2013, http://edition.cnn.com/2013/12/06/world/africa/nelson-mandela-surprising-facts/index.html
3. Albert Steffen, *Kunst als Weg zur Einweihung. Der Künstler als Sozialtherapeut*, Frankfurt am Main, 1984.
4. See for example the information leaflet *Spontanheilung* issued by the Gesellschaft für biologische Krebsabwehr in May 2011.
5. Elise Wolfram/Paracelsus, D*ie Okkulten Ursachen der Krankheiten, Volumen paramirum,* Dornach, 1991.
6. 'Gesundheit heisst, einen kreativen Umgang mit den Grenzen des Könnens zu entwickeln', interview with Professor Giovanni Maio, MD, MA phil., in *Info3*, issue 1/2015, p. 27.
7. Free download at www.gerald huether.de/populaer/audio/alleaudios/?page=1
8. Sir William Osler, *The Principles and Practice of Medicine*, New York, 1947.
9. 'Stellungnahme des Wissenschaftlichen Beirats der Bundesärztekammer "Placebo in der Medizin"', in *Deutsches Ärzteblatt*, 107, issue 28-29, July 2010, p. A1417.
10. Ibid.
11. Bruno Klopfer, 'Psychological variables in human cancer', in *Journal of Projective Techniques,* vol. 21, no. 4 (December 1957), p 331-340.
12. Caryle Hirshberg, Marc Ian Barasch, *Gesund werden aus eigener Kraft. Spontanheilung bei Krebs,* Munich, p. 393ff.
13. For instance, see www.focus.de/wissen/experten/stollmann/von-agelasten-und-gelotophoben-leben-sie-gesund-lachen-sie-sich-tot_id_3873583.html
14. Kurt Langbein, in *Gesundheit Aktiv*, issue 1/2015.
15. See www.eurogrube.de/gesundheit-fitness/regeneration-raucherlunge.htm
16. Steffen Schaal, Konrad Kunsch, Steffen Kunsch, *Der Mensch in Zahlen. Eine Datensammlung in Tabellen mit über 20.000 Einzelwerten*, Stuttgart 2015.
17. Wolfgang Hiddemann, Claus R. Bartram, *Die Onkologie. Epidemiologie, Pathogenese, Grundprinzipien der Therapie,* Berlin, 2004, p. 121.
18. Wolfgang Schad in a panel discussion on the film *Das creative Universum. Naturwissenschaft und Spiritualität im Dialog* (see note 24 above). See www.youtube.com/watch?v=9Sz8o5p8RhI
19. Walter M. Gallmeier, 'Phänomene, die wir nicht erklären können', in *Focus Magazin*, no. 23 (1995).

20. Peter Lahnstein, *Schillers Leben*, Frankfurt am Main 1985, p. 457f.
21. Rudolf Steiner, 'Der Krankheitswahn im Lichte der Geisteswissenschaft', in *Die Erkenntnis der Seele und des Geistes* (GA 56), lecture of 3 December 1907, Dornach 1985, p. 205.
22. See for instance the article by the German cancer research centre at www.krebsinformationsdienst.de/grundlagen/krebsstatistiken.php
23. Rudolf Steiner, 'Der Krankheitswahn im Lichte der Geisteswissenschaft', p. 191.
24. These ideas originated with the anatomist Josef Hyrtl. See H. Christof Müller-Busch, *Abschied braucht Zeit. Palliativmedizin und Ethik des Sterbens*, Frankfurt am Main, 2012.
25. Novalis, 'Neue Fragmente: Von der geheimen Welt', in *Werke und Briefe*, ed. by Alfred Keletat, Stuttgart, p. 454.
26. See books on near-death experiences, including: Raymond A. Moody, *Life after Life*, Rider, 2001; George G. Ritchie, *Return from Tomorrow*, Chosen Books, 2007; Eben Alexander, *Proof of Heaven*, Piatkus, 2012; Rudolf Steiner, *Leben nach dem Tod*, Ausgewählte Texte, Basel, 2008; Anita Moorjani, *Dying to be Me*, Hay House, 2012.
27. The Dalai Lama, quoted in lectures by Carl Simonton.
28. Rudolf Steiner, e.g. in GA 264, *Zur Geschichte und aus den Inhalten der ersten Abteilung der Esoterischen Schule 1904 bis 1914*, Dornach 1996, p. 101. Cf. also Rudolf Steiner, GA 261, *Unsere Toten. Ansprachen, Gedenkworte und Meditationssprüche 1906-1924*, Dornach 1984; or also GA 168, *Die Verbindung zwischen Lebenden und Toten,* Dornach 1995.
29. From a poem by Dietrich Bonhoeffer, in Ruth-Alice von Bismarck, ed. *Brautbriefe Zelle 92. Dietrich Bonhoeffer – Maria Wedemayer 1943-1945*, Munich 1992, p. 208ff.
30. See Grünter Rolling's interview with Elisabeth Kübler-Ross, www.youtube.com/watch?v=C_KHpHlsAM4.
31. André Heller in his lecture of 29 January 2004 in Tübingen.
32. Juan Ramón Jiménez, *Herz, stirb oder singe,* Zurich, 1977.
33. Rudolf Steiner made very extensive, detailed comments on this theme. See for instance, *Das Leben nach dem Tod und sein Zusammenhang mit der Welt der Lebenden*, thirteen lectures, ed. by Frank Teichmann, Stuttgart 2011; Rudolf Steiner, *Leben nach dem Tod*, selected texts, ed. by Hans Stauffer, Basel 2008; Arie Boogert, *Der Weg der Seele nach dem Tod. Unser Leben nach dem Leben*, Stuttgart 2012.
34. Steve Jobs in his Stanford speech on 12 June 2005.
35. Quoted in Lisa Puyplat, *Salvador Dalí: Facetten eines Jahrhundertkünstlers,* Würzburg, 2005, p. 172.
36. Lisa Laurenz, 'Segensreiche Quelle. Über das Mysterium des Herzens', radio broadcast by SWR, 9 April 2012.
37. Ibid.
38. Ibid.
39. Anita Moorjani, *Dying To Be Me,* Hay House 2012.

40. Ibid.
41. Ibid.
42. Ibid.
43. See also Jutta Richter, *An einem grossen stillen See*, Munich 2003.
44. Steve Jobs in his Stanford speech on 12 June 2005.
45. From an Arte TV documentary on Christoph Schlingensief.
46. See www.grossarth-maticek.de/seiten/frame_forschung.html
47. Aaron Antonovsky, *Salutogenese. Zur Entmystifizierung der Gesundheit,* Tübingen, 1997.
48. From the film *Die Heilkraft des inneren Arztes* by Sabine Goette.
49. Gerald Hüther in his foreword to the book by Otto Teischel, *Krankheit und Sehnsucht – Zur Psychosomatik der Sucht. Hintergründe – Symptome – Heilungswege,* Heidelberg, 2014, p. vii.
50. Ibid, p. IX.
51. David Servan-Schreiber, *Das Anti-Krebs-Buch. Was uns schützt: Vorbeugen und Nachsorgen mit natürlichen Mitteln,* Augsburg 2009.
52. Pablo Picasso, Wort und Bekenntnis, Frankfurt, 1957, p. 19.
53. A wonderful book for studying this in detail is: Marshall B. Rosenberg, *Nonviolent Communication: A Language of Life,* PuddleDancer Press 2015.
54. George G. Ritchie, *Return from Tomorrow*, Chosen Books, 2007.
55. From a lecture by Anselm Grün in Bad Herrenhalb, Germany, 2008.
56. The Dalai Lama in his foreword to the book *The Tibetan Book of Living and Dying,* Harper Collins, 1992.
57. From a lecture by Sabine Mehne, co-founder of the 'Near-Death Experience Network', Mühltal, Germany, which she gave on 30 January 2011 with cardiologist Pim van Lommel, co-founder of the Dutch section of the International Association for Near-Death Studies.
58. Novalis, journal entry for 9 October 1800 in *Werke und Briefe*, ed. by Alfred Kelletat, Stuttgart, p. 700.
59. Cf. Gerald Hüther in his lecture *Die Neurobiologie des Glücks* and in the radio broadcast *SWR2Wissen: Aula* on 4 December 2011.
60. Antonio Machado in *Lands of Castile and Other Poems,* Liverpool University Press 2002.
61. Interview with Gunver Kienle MD in *Gesundheit Aktiv*, issue 02/2–15, p. 34.
62. Cf. Rudolf Steiner, *Seelenübungen* vol. I (GA 267), Dornach, 2001, p. 87.
63. Lawrence LeShan, *Diagnose Krebs, Wendepunkt und Neubeginn. Ein Handbuch für Menschen, die an Krebs leiden, für ihre Familien und ihre Ärzte und Therapeuten,* Stuttgart, 2013.
64. Christoph Schlingensief, *Ich weiss, ich war's*, ed. by Aino Laberenz, Munich, 2014.
65. Johann Wolfgang von Goethe, 'Maximen und Reflexionen' in *Werke*, vol. 12, Hamburg, 1994, p. 443.
66. From a talk by the Nobel judge Claes Gustafsson on 7 October 2015.

67. 'Gesundheit heisst, einen kreativen Umgang mit den Grenzen des Könnens zu entwickeln', interview with Professor Giovanni Maio, MD, MA phil., in *Info3*, issue 1/2015, p. 27.
68. Julia Friedrichs, 'Der Preis der Hoffnung', in *Zeitmagazin*, no. 2/2016, 7 January 2016. See also www.zeit.de/zeit-magazin/2016/02/medikamente-krebs-hexavar-markt-neuheit-risiko
69. Christian Schubert in the foreword to *Psychoneuroimmunologie und Psychotherapie*, 2nd edn, Stuttgart, 2015.

Acknowledgements

Thanks to the publishers and copyright holders below for their kind permission to reprint the following works.

Hilde Domin, 'Es gibt dich', from *Gesammelte Gedichte* S. Fischer Verlag GmbH, Frankfurt am Main, 1987.

Erich Fried, 'Was es ist', from *Es ist was es ist* Verlag Klaus Wagenbach, Berlin, 1983.

Dag Hammarskjöld, *Markings*, Faber and Faber, 1988.

Sabine Mehne, 'Neu in den Füssen stehn' from *Licht ohne Schatten. Leben mit einer Nahtoderfahrung* Patmos Verlag in der Schwabenverlag AG Ostfildern, 3rd edition 2013, www.verlagsgruppe-patmos.de

Christian Morgenstern, 'Was wärst du, Wind' from *Werke und Briefe,* vol. II, *Lyrik 1906-1914*, ed. by Martin Kiessig, Stuttgart, 1992.

Jutta Richter, 'Der Neinengel' from *An einem grossen stillen See*, illustrated by Susanne Jenssen-Mechler, Carl Hanser Verlag, Munich, 2003.

Rudolf Steiner, 'Ergebensheitgebet' from *Pfade der Seelenerlebnisse* (GA 59), lecture of 17 February 1910, 'Das Wesen des Gebetes', Dornach, 2002.

Rudolf Steiner, 'Ich trage Ruhe in mir' from *Mantrische Sprüche, Seelenübungen*, vol. II, 1903–1925 (GA 268), Dornach, 2015.